A Concise International History of Rheumatology and Rehabilitation

Friends and Foes

George D Kersley and John Glyn

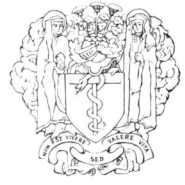

Royal Society of Medicine Services Limited

Royal Society of Medicine Services Limited
1 Wimpole Street London W1M 8AE
8 East 60th Street New York NY 10022

© 1991 Royal Society of Medicine Services Limited

Apart from any fair dealing for the purposes of research or private study, or criticism or review, as permitted under the Copyright, Designs and Patents Act, 1988, no part of this publication may be reproduced, stored, or transmitted, in any form or by any means, without the prior permission in writing of the publishers, or in the case of reprographic reproduction in accordance with the terms of licences issued by the Copyright Licensing Agency in the UK, or in accordance with the terms of licences issued by the appropriate Reproduction Rights Organization outside the UK. Enquiries concerning reproduction outside the terms stated here should be sent to the publishers at the above address.

British Library Cataloguing in Publication Data

Kersley, G. D.
   A concise international history of rheumatology and
   rehabilitation—friends and foes.
   1. Man. Joints. Arthritis & rheumatic diseases
   I. Title II. Glyn, J.
   616.72

   ISBN 1-85315-141-6
   ISBN 1-85315-140-8 (pbk)

The authors are responsible for the historical and scientific content of this book.

Editorial and production services by Diane Crofter Harris

Phototypeset by Dobbie Typesetting Limited, Tavistock, Devon

Printed in Great Britain by Henry Ling

Contents

List of Illustrations		vi
Foreword		ix
Introduction		xi
Chapter 1	**The Beginnings**	1
	Hydrotherapy and the Spas	1
	The Spas	1
	La Ligue Contre le Rhumatism	9
	Subsequent Leagues Against Rheumatism	12
	The International League ILAR	14
	The Continental Leagues	14
	The British League	17
	Early Physiotherapy	18
Chapter 2	**The 1930s**	21
	The Clinical Picture	21
	Orthopaedics	23
	The Beginning of Rheumatology	25
	Participants in the Beginning of Rheumatology in the UK	31
	The Royal College of Physicians	31
	The Empire Rheumatism Council (ERC, ARC)	31
	Peto Place and the Arthur Stanley Institute	34
	The Heberden Society	35
	The Royal Society of Medicine (RSM)	42
	The Charterhouse Clinic	42
	Our Hospitals in the 1930s	43
Chapter 3	**The War Years**	45
	The British Association of Physical Medicine (BAPM)	48
Chapter 4	**The Post-War Period and the National Health Service**	51
	The National Health Service	51
	Internecine War—Two Views	54
	1940-1950 (GDK)	54
	1949-1990 (JG)	56

Chapter	**5 Participants in Post-War Developments**	65
	Hospital Developments	65
	The Canadian Red Cross Hospital, Taplow	65
	The Kennedy Institute	65
	The Spinal Injuries Centre, Stoke Mandeville	66
	Patient Involvement	67
	The British Rheumatism Association (Arthritis Care)	68
	The Horder Homes	68
	The Back Pain Association and Society	69
	British Association of Manipulative Medicine	69
	The National Osteoporosis Society	70
	The National Ankylosing Spondylitis Society	70
	Other Groups	70
Chapter	**6 American Rheumatology and Physiatry**	71
	Developments in the USA	71
	Rheumatology	71
	Physiatry	74
Chapter	**7 The Evolution and Spectrum of Rheumatic Diseases 1930-1990**	77
	Rheumatic Fever	77
	Some Reasons for the Expanding Spectrum	77
	Immunopathology and Rheumatology	78
	Endocrine and Metabolic Diseases	78
	Methods of Investigation	78
	'New' and Newly Interpreted Diseases	78
	Non-rheumatic Diseases Presenting with Skeletal Pains	79
	Eclectic Case Loads	79
	Medical Orthopaedics	80
	Prophylactic, Salvage and Replacement Surgery	80
	Sports Medicine	80
	Rehabilitation	80
	Electrodiagnosis	81
	References	81
Chapter	**8 Evolution and Spectrum of Drug Therapy**	83
	Pre-War to the 1950s	83
	References	84
	1949-1990	84
	Corticosteroids	84

Non-Steroidal Anti-Inflammatory Drugs	85
Phenylbutazones	86
Indomethacin and later NSAIDs	87
Disease Modifying Drugs	88
Anti-Malarial Drugs in Rheumatology	88
D-Penicillamine	89
Sulphasalazine	89
Local Use of Anti-Proliferative Drugs	90
Immunosuppression	91
More Recent Developments in the Management of Gout	91
Xanthine Oxidase Inhibition	91
References	92

Chapter 9 The Evolution of Rehabilitation — 93
Specialised Rehabilitation — 96

Chapter 10 The Evolution and Process of Fusion — 99
Recent Developments — 100

Chapter 11 Epilogue — 103

Biographies — 105

Appendices — 127
Meetings and Presidents of the Leagues — 127
British Association of Physical Medicine (BAPM), later The British Association for Rheumatology and Rehabilitation (BARR) — 129
British Society for Rheumatology (BSR) — 129
Presidents, Orators and Roundsmen of the Heberden Society — 130
Some Important Dates in the History of British Rheumatology and Rehabilitation — 134
Notes on the History of Units in the UK with Professorial Chairs in Rheumatology and Rehabilitation — 136

Index — 143

Addendum — 150

List of Illustrations

George Kersley — back cover

John Glyn — back cover

Cranach's painting of 'The Fountain of Youth'. 1546, Berlin. (Staatliche Museum, Berlin) — 2

Dr Oliver and Mr Peirce—the first medico-surgical consultation, 1742. (Royal National Hospital for Rheumatic Diseases) — 2

Bath Spa, 1675. — 3

British Spas Federation Dinner at Bath, May 1957. — 4

Conference Dinner at the Annual Conference of the British Spas Federation at Buxton, May 1951. — 5

Some council members of the International Society of Medical Hydrology at their annual meeting in Hungary, 1929. (Eric Bywaters) — 7

International Society of Medical Hydrology, Dinner, 1946. — 8

International Committee for the Study of Rheumatology, 1927, with Mussolini in the centre. — 9

Anthem composed by Van Breemen for La Ligue Internationale Contre le Rhumatism. — 10

La Ligue Contre le Rhumatism at Malmo, Dinner, 1936. — 11

Jacques Forestier. (Eric Bywaters) — 12

Fortescue Fox. (Eric Bywaters) — 13

J Van Breemen. (Eric Bywaters) — 13

Ralph Pemberton. — 14

Honorary Members of the American Rheumatism Association elected to celebrate the first meeting of the International League held in New York, 1949. — 15

List of Illustrations

Meeting in New York at which the International League Against Rheumatism was formed, Dinner, 1949.	16
Professor Nesterov. (Eric Bywaters)	17
Sir John Charnley.	24
Lord Horder. (Eric Bywaters)	27
Will Copeman. (Elizabeth Dawson)	28
Empire Rheumatism Council, 21st Birthday Celebration, 1947. Guests at the top table.	32
All Branches meeting of ARC. George Kersley, Mrs Pryor (Bath representative), Rt Hon Hornsby-Smith (Vice-Chairman ARC), Colin G Barnes (Chairman ARC Scientific Committee).	34
Phillip Hench.	36
Wine list signed by committee members of the Heberden Society, 1947.	37
William Heberden. (Ernest Heberden, from *William Heberden*, Royal Society of Medicine Services, 1989.)	38
Seven Heberden Presidents, 1979. Michael Andrews (Secretary), Eric Bywaters, John Ball, Allan Dixon, Leonard Glynn, 'Frank' Dudley Hart, Tom Scott, George Kersley.	39
Morris Ziff. (Eric Bywaters)	40
Physical Medicine Section, Royal Society of Medicine Dinner, 1941.	41
The British Army Physical Medicine Team, 1942.	45
Col George Kersley, 1942, Adviser in Physical Medicine to Middle East.	46
FD Howitt CVO, President of the Heberden Society. Leader of the Physical Medicine Team.	47
Signed menu of a meeting of the British Association of Physical Medicine, 1945.	49

First International Congress of Physical Medicine, 1952.   50

Heberden Society Dinner, 1962 at the House of Commons.   54

Professor Eric Bywaters.   66

Professor Jonas Kellgren.   67

Currier McEwen. (Eric Bywaters)   73

Joseph Hollander. (Eric Bywaters)   85

The progeny of some of the more commonly used   86
non-steroidal anti-inflammatory drugs.

The last Heberden Society Annual Dinner and Foundation   101
Dinner of the British Society of Rheumatology, 1983.

Foreword

There are two good reasons why I am happy to write the Foreword to this excellent little book. The first is that one of the authors is an old friend of mine and as one grows older these become correspondingly more valuable. The second is that I was privileged, with him, to see the launching of the Empire Rheumatism Council (the forerunner of the Arthritis and Rheumatism Council), some fifty years ago. It was a prestigious birth—held at St James's Palace—with the then Duke of Gloucester as President, Lord Horder the Royal Physician as Chairman and Sir William Willcox, the eminent forensic physician of the day, as Chairman of the Scientific Advisory Committee. Horder was the power behind the throne in the formation of rheumatology as a respectable specialty and, through the British Association of Physical Medicine, also of rehabilitation. Dr WSC Copeman was the first 'rheumatologist' to be recognised as such by the Royal College of Physicians and Dr George Kersley (co-author of this book) was the second in this field. Let us not forget that at that time the whole group of the rheumatic diseases was nothing but the 'waste-paper basket' of general medicine. Dr John Glyn's experiences related to training and practising within a divided profession in the post-war period.

As an orthopaedic surgeon manqué, I have maintained a life-long interest in bones and joints—hence again it was a great privilege for me, on my retirement, to serve first as Chairman and then, until quite lately, as President of the Arthritis and Rheumatism Council.

I have therefore found this book instructive, informative, interesting and comprehensive. As the authors so modestly say, it is not intended to compete with the erudite and more lengthy publications on various aspects of the subject. It is a 'concise history' of both International and British Rheumatology in all its aspects, including the effect of the National Health Service and the wars on these. It achieves something that none of its contemporaries do—it stresses the increasing symbiosis between rheumatology and rehabilitation—a concept of major importance in today's medical world. When one realises the enormity and the significance of the rheumatic diseases as the greatest cause of human suffering and of economic loss in the whole range of medicine, it is obvious that this little book is indeed timely. There are times when it is good to look back and count our blessings; this book does so—and I wish it well.

The Rt Hon Lord Porritt, GCVO, CBE, FRCS, FRCP

Introduction

Rehabilitation in some form goes back to antiquity, though initially it was concerned more with fitness, the body beautiful, attempted postponement of senescence and promotion of fecundity. The wars, certainly back to the Crimea, have added some stimulus to its study.

Erudite histories of the Heberden Society and the Arthritis and Rheumatism Council and a chronicle of the British Association of Physical Medicine, outlining the history of modern rehabilitation, have recently been or are in the process of being written. Until now however, no concise history has brought rheumatology and rehabilitation together and shown the effects of one on the other.

This book gives a brief history of all the factors and societies, medical and lay, that have played a part in building up the specialties of rheumatology and rehabilitation as we know them today.

It also gives the views and problems as seen by one of the earliest rheumatologists, who temporarily, owing to World War II, became a physical medicine specialist, George Kersley, and a younger physician, John Glyn, who was caught up in the post-war battles between the two specialties.

Certain sections have been written by one or other authors, expressing his views and therefore he has repeated previously recorded facts in order to substantiate slants on how he saw problems and how they were resolved. Again there may be slight overlap between the early history of therapy and the subsequent role of drug treatment in shaping rheumatology today. Any reiteration has however been kept to a minimum.

The story shows the effect of the war and subsequently of the National Health Service (NHS) on these problems and how they have gradually been solved. In addition to the situation in the UK, the evolution of rheumatology and physical medicine on the Continent and in the USA has also been briefly recorded.

A section of short biographies of those who have greatly contributed to both rheumatology and physical medicine is included. An Appendix lists the names and dates of all the Presidents of the Leagues against Rheumatism, of the Heberden Society and its Orators and of the Presidents of the British Association of Physical Medicine. There is also a list of dates of importance, such as the establishment of Chairs in Rheumatology.

This is the first book to record briefly the history of both specialties, going back to their earliest roots; it is intended to be for easy reference. Included are anecdotal passages about events never yet described and which throw light on why some problems arose and how they were solved, and also personal experiences that illustrate the changes that have come about in both specialties during the last half century.

In 1932 George Kersley was accused by Professor Sir Francis Fraser of 'prostituting his soul' if he joined the 'quacks' in even part-time specialising in rheumatology. Some seventeen years later John Glyn met with a somewhat similar reaction from his chief, Professor Alan Kekwick, and was embroiled as a young post-war would-be consultant in the search for a niche in rheumatology and/or physical medicine.

Rheumatology took some twenty years to become established, undoubtedly helped by the discovery of cortisone by a rheumatologist, Phil Hench. As Lord Horder expressed it, 'The Princes of Medicine [the academics] finally recognised Cinderella [rheumatology] at the Ball'.

Having done much, as part of the war effort, to establish physical medicine temporarily, those previously involved in the treatment and research into arthritis were most anxious that their status should not be dragged down again by a new specialty, in which many members were less well qualified. On the other hand those recently recruited to physical medicine were most anxious for rheumatology and rehabilitation to become synonymous, thus gaining them access to hospital beds and private practice.

The Department of Health and Social Security (DHSS) added to the confusion by calling the registrars in rheumatology, trainees in physical medicine, and it took all the influence of the College of Physicians and that great catholic-minded physician, Lord Horder, who took the lead in establishing both specialties, to pour oil on the troubled waters.

Let us now, however, return to the beginnings.

Chapter 1

The Beginnings

Hydrotherapy and the spas
It all started with hydrology. Even in 2000 BC in Babylonia the words *A Su* connected water with healing. In Roman times the baths were the centre for treatment, but also culture and sometimes debauchery. At Ephesus a brothel was incorporated. It was however in the 18th century that spa treatment became of real importance, though in the previous century it was used extensively to promote fertility and fecundity—witness Cranach's lovely painting of the sick and aged discarding their crutches on one side of the pool and pairing off in the undergrowth on the other side (page 2).

The Spas
In the UK, as on the Continent, rheumatology was first centred on the spas. Most of the early books dealing with arthritis and gout were written by the great spa physicians, many of whom also practised in London and elsewhere out of the spa season. The spa physicians, George Cheyne in 1720 and William Oliver in 1751 wrote important monographs on gout; in 1889 Dr J Spender added his work on osteoarthritis and in 1896 GA Bannatyne produced a valuable paper on rheumatoid arthritis.

Not surprisingly, the major hospitals for the treatment of rheumatic disease grew up around the spas. At Bath the only hot spring waters in the country were valued for occult and religious purposes in pre-Roman times, but in 45 AD, as *Aquae Sulis*, the famous baths were constructed for treatment, relaxation, beauty therapy, at times debauchery and as a centre for debates and teaching. The great Roman physician Galen had advised balneotherapy for treatment of joints and the urinary tract. After the departure of the Romans, the baths collapsed into a swamp and the waters became the property of the church till the 16th century when they were handed over to the City. It was however a hundred years later that spas in England and on the Continent began to be again used for treatment, the 18th and 19th centuries being their heyday.

In 1742 the Bath Hospital (later the Royal Mineral Water Hospital and now the Royal National Hospital for Rheumatic Diseases) was established for 150 sick poor from outside the city. It was enlarged in 1861. It is the oldest hospital in the world to be devoted to the treatment of arthritis. The analysis of the diagnoses of admissions

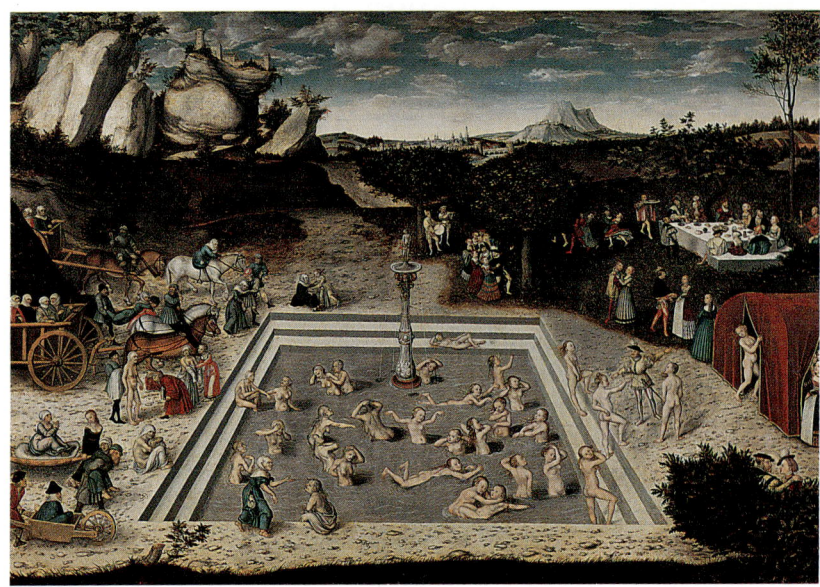

Cranach's painting of 'The Fountain of Youth', 1546, Berlin. (Staatliche Museum, Berlin)

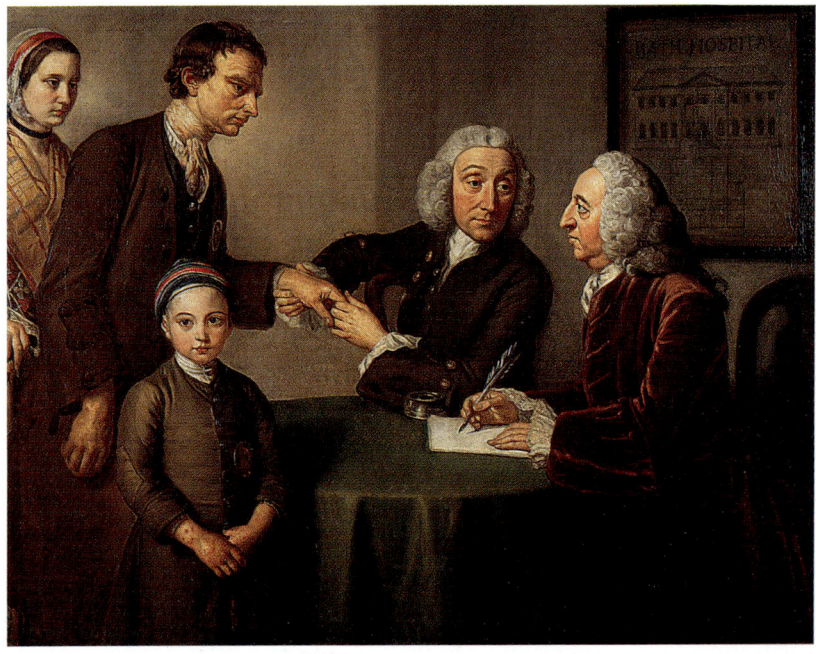

Dr Oliver and Mr Peirce—the first medico-surgical consultation, 1742. (Royal National Hospital for Rheumatic Diseases)

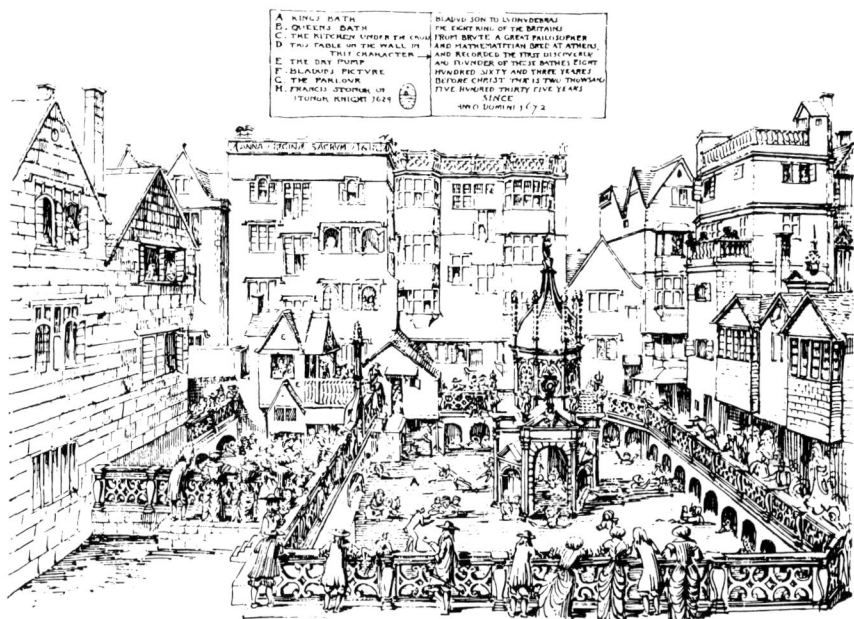

Bath Spa, 1675.

to the Bath Hospital show that in 1760 only 26% were recorded as rheumatic with the remainder mostly paralytic (40%) while many other patients were admitted for skin conditions. By 1860, however, the number of cases of 'rheumatism', including sciatica, had risen to 62% with many of the remainder diagnosed as lead palsy. In 1936 a new hospital of 220 beds with an orthopaedic department was authorised, but war intervened and after many difficulties and struggles with a series of governments, the old hospital, apart from the addition of a research floor, was modernised within the original buildings. It was reopened by Princess Marina in 1965. There are now 100 beds.

Even before the foundation of the Bath Hospital, Bellotts Hospital was built in 1611, not just as a rest house like most 'hospitals' of that time, but for twelve patients from outside Bath for the treatment of locomotor disease. Only in London (St Bartholomew's and St Thomas's) are there any older foundations that were established for serious treatment rather than as hospices.

At Buxton the warm springs were used by the Romans as *Aquae Arnemethiae* until the Romans left the country. Then in the 16th century under the patronage of the Earl of Shrewsbury the waters began to be used again. The Royal Devonshire Hospital was built in 1858, when the Duke of Devonshire's stables, built in 1798 for 110 horses, were reconstructed. Much of the impetus came from the Buxton Bath Charity founded in 1572: treatment was restricted to patients from beyond a seven mile radius. In 1881 it was expanded

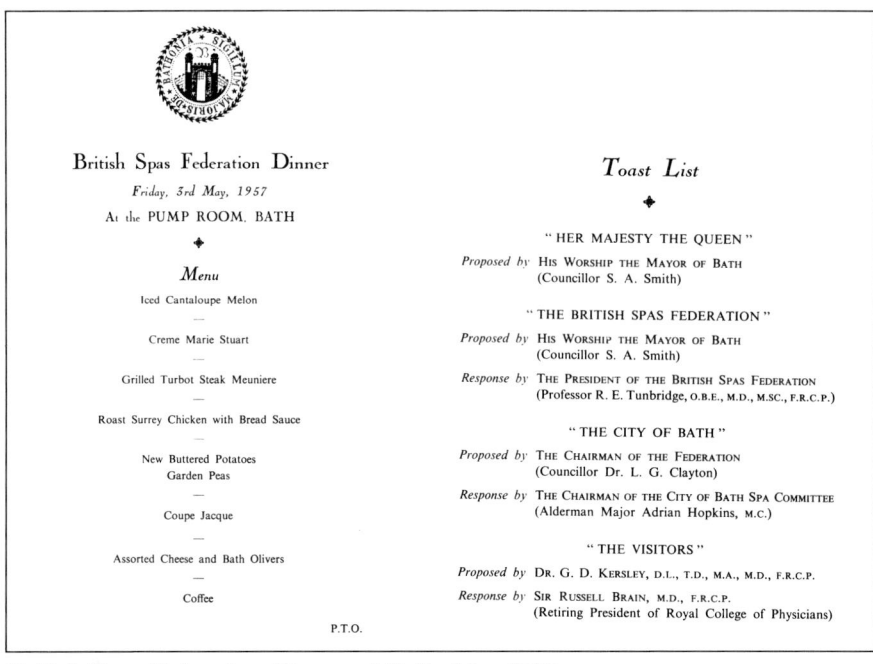

British Spas Federation Dinner at Bath, May 1957.

and the largest dome in the world at that time was built to roof the central exercising ground of the original stables. There were 230 beds. This is now reduced to 163: 68 for rheumatology, 65 for rehabilitation and 30 for orthopaedics.

At Harrogate the sulphurous waters were not discovered till the 17th century and the baths not opened till 1897. In 1826 the Royal Bath Hospital at Harrogate, for patients living outside a three mile radius, was opened on Lord Harewood's land. This facility was largely due to the efforts of a Trust for Relief of the Poor, founded some fifty years earlier. The hospital had 130 beds, including 33 orthopaedic, but is now reduced to 70 beds. The Rawson Convalescent Centre was run in close liaison with this hospital, but in 1924 became a research laboratory and is now an attached Clinical Pharmacology Unit.

Other establishments predominantly treating the rheumatic diseases were at Droitwich, known to the Romans as a source of salt, but where the waters were not used medicinally till 1830 when they were employed for the treatment of a cholera epidemic; Royal Leamington Spa dates from 1814 and received the title of Royal from the patronage of Queen Victoria.

Seawater bathing for arthritic conditions, and especially tubercular diseases of bone, was sponsored by Sir Henry Gauvain who had much to do with the founding of the orthopaedic hospital at Alton.

To these major spa hospitals were added the rheumatology beds at St Stephen's Hospital, London and at St John and St Elizabeth

Hospital, London in 1937 and the West London Rheumatology Department in 1938.

In the early part of this century there were many other spas in England, Scotland and Wales. Nineteen are listed in the Spas Federation Handbook of 1919, but only six in 1951.

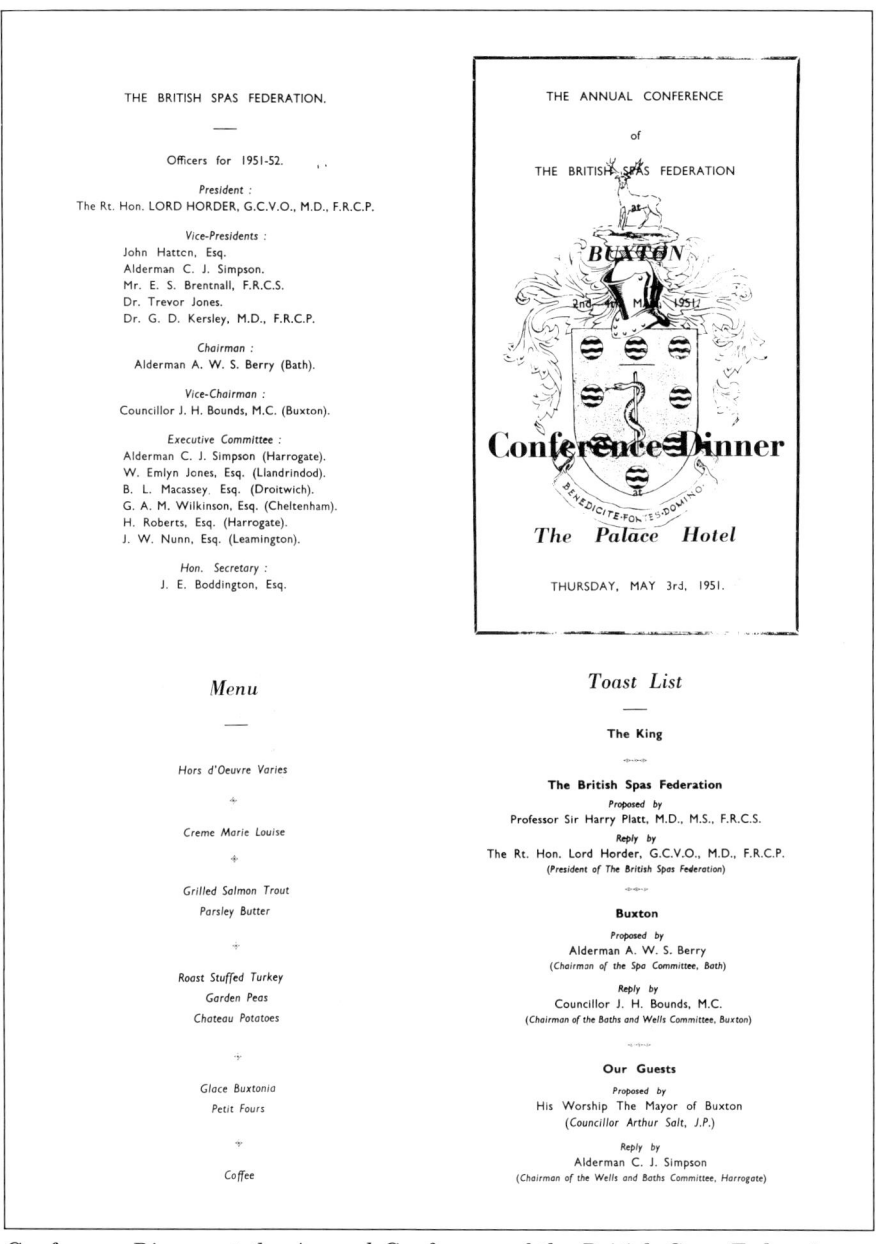

Conference Dinner at the Annual Conference of the British Spas Federation at Buxton, May 1951.

Outside the UK, spas have continued to flourish, except in Scandinavia and the USA. In France, spa therapy is part of the medical training of every doctor and such treatment is a right under their social security system, though the right to claim the cost of travel and accommodation depends on the patient's means. Five of the largest spas belong to the State and the remainder to private enterprise. About three-quarters of the patients are supported by social security.

In West Germany, spa popularity has gone to the extreme, costing 2% of the gross national product. In 1975 there were over six million visitors officially going for treatment and of these nearly half a million were foreign. The spa industry is flourishing so greatly that in Baden Baden they are currently building 24 new hotels to cope with the influx.

Behind the 'Iron Curtain', spas are also well used and proliferating, filled by state financed clientele, both for treatment and for health-giving holidays, and they are also now becoming useful earners of foreign currency.

Lately, political considerations have influenced the spas in Eastern Europe very greatly. Though always of importance, partly for treatment and partly as a health giving reward for good service of 'nationals', in Hungary, which has always wanted closer contact and friendship with the West, even before 'Glasnost', they have opened up or refurbished six major spas with great success, entirely to cater for and gain currency from Western Europe and the USA. This is in addition to nearly a hundred smaller spas, run by the Health Service or Trades Unions for Hungarians. In Czechoslovakia, however, there has been, one hopes temporarily, the opposite reaction, the Government discouraging 'foreigners' from coming for treatment. This is particularly disappointing as much good work has been carried out in that country by such enthusiasts as Lenoch and more recently Sitaj. Happily, however, that situation is now changing.

At Bath, the spa closed in 1976 when the NHS withdrew its support. This was a matter of economy, as there were hydrotherapy facilities at the Royal National Hospital for Rheumatic Disease and the Royal United Hospital. The City is now handing it over to private enterprise. It is the only natural hot water spa in the UK and this led to a problem in the use of the waters when in 1978 a girl died of amoebic meningitis after swimming in a bath fed from the spring. It was discovered that an amoeba, *Naegleriae fowleri*, that could exist in a resistant cystic form, had been found in pooled hot water in many parts of the world. If inhaled it could reach the brain via the sinuses and then cause fatal meningitis. In Bath there was near to panic and many thought dipping a foot in the water would cause certain death. After consultation with Dr Paul Mann, our public health expert, I said it was even safe to drink, if not inhaled. On being challenged, I then drank a large tumbler during a televised interview, but when they wanted a retake, I said only if the second tumbler was laced with whisky! Since then two further thermophilic amoebae have been discovered, but these are not pathogenic to human beings—though one is to mice! The experts on geological strata and engineering have since drilled a shaft to tap the fault through which the water came to the surface well below the silt where the amoebae were flourishing. A pure supply of the hot water has therefore now been obtained.

The obvious value of the spas is for rehabilitation with an accent on hydrotherapy, but, combined with all other appropriate treatment, it is carried out in an atmosphere free from stress and with a bonus of the engendered patient's belief and hope. Interest in the British spas is again increasing, but with a definite element of recreation and facilities for the provision of better health and fitness.

During the war the spas dealt with rehabilitation of the wounded. When the NHS came into being I (GDK) was asked to represent their case to Lord Horder, Sir Wilson Jamieson, Sir Adolph Abrahams and Sir Henry, later Lord Cohen. After being rebuked by Horder, my old chief, for not mentioning the value of belief and hope in the use of the 'waters', it was agreed that the NHS could pay for patients' rehabilitation at the spas on prescription of a consultant. Patients were asked 'Do you wish to pay or have the treatment free?'—95% therefore came through the NHS.

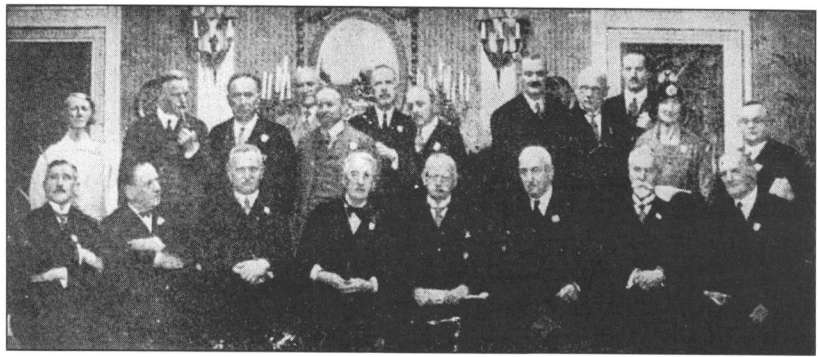

Some council members of the International Society of Medical Hydrology at their annual meeting in Hungary, 1929. (Eric Bywaters)
Front Row (left to right): Prof Gunzburg (Belgium, representing Dr Wybauw), Senatore Prof Gabbi (Italy), Prof Strasser (Austria), Dr Fortescue Fox (Chairman), Ministerialdirektor Prof Dr Dietrich (Germany), Dr Fodor (Austria), Prof Wateff (Bulgaria), Dr Van Breemen (Holland). Back row: Miss Thompson (General Secretary), Dr Arne Faber (Denmark, representing Dr Jansen), Prof Gozzi (Italy, representing Prof Vinaj), Dr Max Wassermann (Czechoslovakia), Dr Mougeot (France), Dr Buckley (Chairman of Finance Committee), Dr Ferreyrolles (France), Dr Burt (England), Dr Taipale (Finland), Dr Copeman (Joint Hon Secretary), Miss Hilda Fox (late Assistant Hon Secretary), Dr Hirsch (Germany).

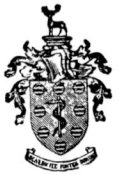

International Society of Medical Hydrology

Buxton, England, October 4th—6th, 1946.
Dinner at the Spa Hotel, Buxton.
Friday, October 4th, 1946, at 8 p.m.

MENU

Hors D'oeuvres
Petit Marmite

Creme a la Reine
Filet de Sole a la Cardinal
ou
Contre Filet de Bœuf Nicoise
ou
Poulet Saute Grande Mere

Choux de Bruxelles
Pommes Fondantes

Glace Vanille
Crepe au Confiiture
Cafe

TOASTS

1. "The International Society of Medical Hydrology."
   Proposed by Councillor J. H. Bounds, M.C., J.P.
   (Mayor of Buxton).
   Replied to by Lord Horder, G.C.V.O., M.D., F.R.C.P.
   (President of the Society).
2. Our Colleagues from Overseas."
   Proposed by Dr. J. Barnes Burt, M.D.
   (Chairman of the Society).
   Replied to by a Delegate from Overseas.

After the Toasts Lord Horder will deliver the Presidential Address.

International Society of Medical Hydrology, Dinner, 1946.

As a matter of economy where other NHS rehabilitation centres were available—the exception being Harrogate which 'opted out' to become a conference centre and upstage dormitory town—this support was gradually withdrawn. The spas were in a parlous state.

The leagues against Rheumatism

La Ligue Contre le Rhumatism

In 1913 at the Physical Medicine Congress in Berlin, Van Breemen, an intrepid and tireless Dutchman, advocated an international league to fight rheumatism. This was not achieved, however, until 1925.

The International Society of Medical Hydrology (ISMH) was founded at a meeting in London by Dr Fortescue Fox with Miss Tatham Thompson as Secretary. It published the *Archives of Medical Hydrology* from 1922 to 1939. In 1925 in Paris, the Committee for the Study of Rheumatology was formed as a branch of ISMH, at the behest of Van Breemen. The original committee consisted of Fox (London), Chairman; Dietrich (Berlin) and Forestier (Paris and Aix les Bains), Vice-Chairmen; Van Breemen (Amsterdam), Secretary General; Gunzburg (Antwerp), Lennep (Amsterdam), Jansen (Copenhagen), Kahlmeter (Stockholm), Korman (Lugano), Schmidt (Piestany), Strasser (Vienna) and Vincent Coates (Bath). This Committee for the Study of Rheumatology met in Prague and then Rome, where Mussolini attended the opening session. In 1928 at its meeting in Buxton it was agreed that the Committee for the Study of Rheumatology should become the nucleus of La Ligue Contre le Rhumatism, which first met in Budapest the next year. Fox retired as President of La Ligue Contre le Rhumatism in 1938, and was succeeded by Ralph Pemberton of Philadelphia.

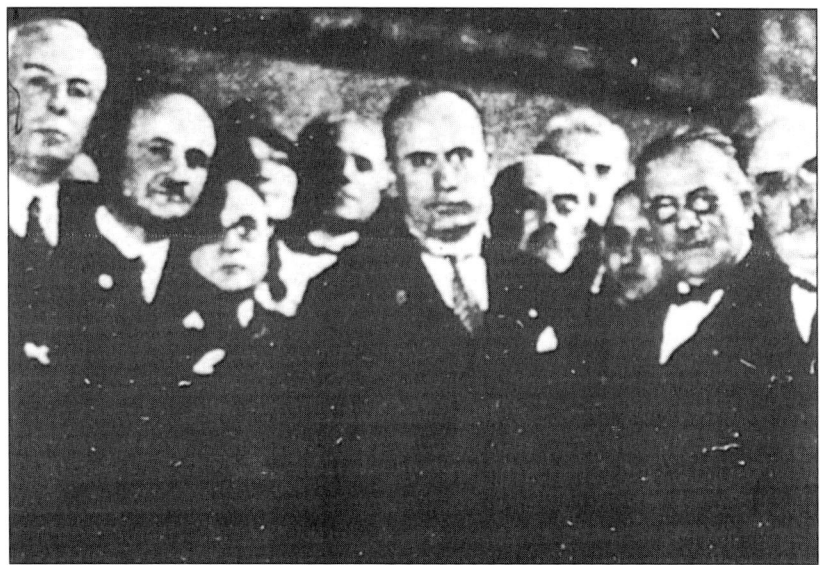

International Committee for the Study of Rheumatology, 1927, with Mussolini in the centre.

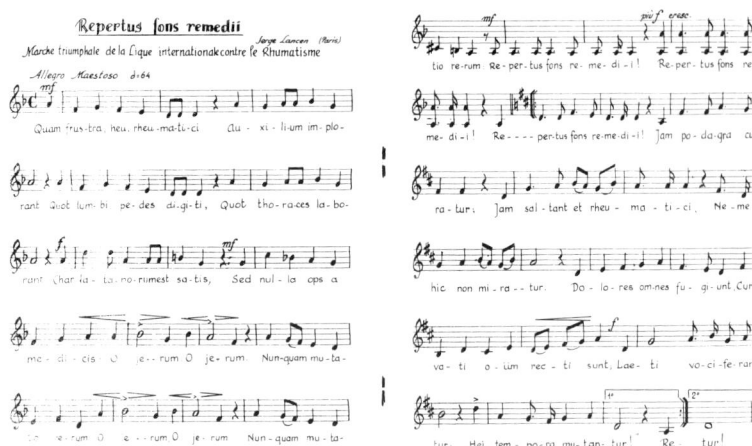

Anthem composed by Van Breemen for La Ligue Internationale Contre le Rhumatism.

La Ligue's objectives were: (1) to act as a central and consultation body in an international campaign against rheumatism; (2) to encourage and assist in the foundation of national committees against rheumatism, without encroaching on their individual liberties or fields of administration; (3) to prepare and circulate general information, statistics and other material.

Meetings were held at Budapest, Vienna, Liege and Paris with meetings at Lund and Stockholm in 1936, and Oxford and Bath in 1938. From 1929 to 1939 the *Acta Rheumatologica* was published. Then everything went into cold storage for the duration of the war.

Professor Gunzburg of Antwerp, who had been President for the meeting in Liege, was imprisoned by the Germans who burnt his house down, destroying many Ligue documents.

All committee work was conducted in French with no interpreter and one had to rely on multilingual friends, like Jacques Forestier, to help one out when one got into difficulties. After the war, with pressure from the Americans and Scandinavians, English began to take precedence, with French second and Spanish third, which suited the South Americans.

The three men who played outstanding parts in La Ligue during these early days, Fox, Van Breemen and Pemberton, could be considered the originators of international rheumatology.

Robert Fortescue Fox was born in 1858, the sixth generation of a line of Quaker doctors, with six brothers who were all doctors. He was father of TF Fox, who became Editor of the *Lancet*. He trained at the London Hospital, but developed tuberculosis and therefore took up a post at Strathpeffer Spa. In World War I he became interested in the rehabilitation of soldiers, and later founded the

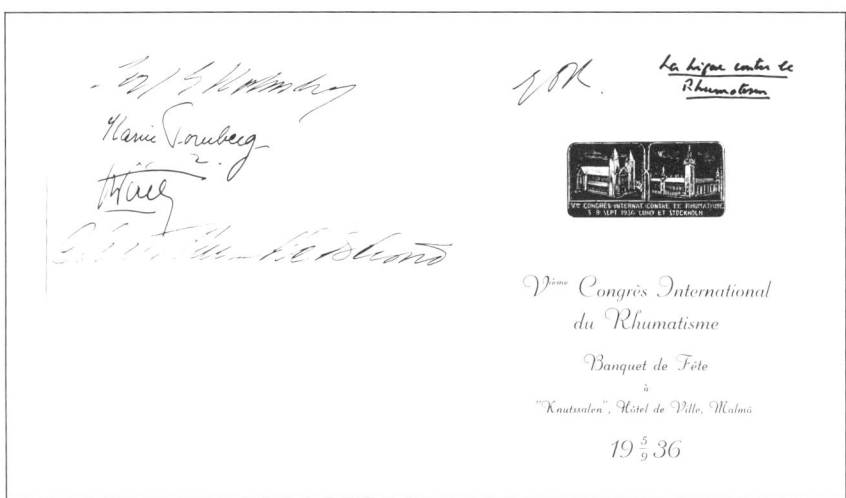

La Ligue contre le Rhumatism at Malmo, 1936.

Enham Village Centre and took a leading part in the start of the Peto Place Red Cross Clinic for Rheumatic Disease. He was Founder Chairman of the ISMH in 1921 and of the Committee for the Study of Rheumatology formed in 1925. He was Editor of the *Archives of Medical Hydrology* and wrote several books on both spa treatment and rehabilitation in arthritis, one on the *Causation and Treatment of Chronic Rheumatism* with Van Breemen. He died in 1940 at the age of 82, having with Van Breemen done more to promote rheumatology and rehabilitation in the 1920s, than any other physician.

J Van Breemen was born in 1873 in Holland and in his early medical career became interested in physical medicine. In 1905 he played a large part in the formation of the Society of Physical Therapy. Though he had the opportunity of building up a huge wealthy private practice, he devoted himself mainly to care of the poor and the organisation of the development of rheumatology from rehabilitation. He first opened the Keizersgracht in Amsterdam for physical treatment of the less well off and did much scientific work to prove or disprove the value of such therapy. He saw at the clinic so many rheumatic patients that his interest veered in that direction. As previously mentioned, he was the driving force behind establishing the Committee for the Study of Rheumatology, the precursor of La Ligue.

Van Breemen edited the *Acta Rheumatologica*, published in three languages. He wrote many books on the aetiology, diagnosis and treatment of chronic rheumatic disease. In 1950 he set to work on establishing the International Research Centre for Rheumatic Disease in Amsterdam, the first centre of its kind in the world. He died in 1960 aged 87.

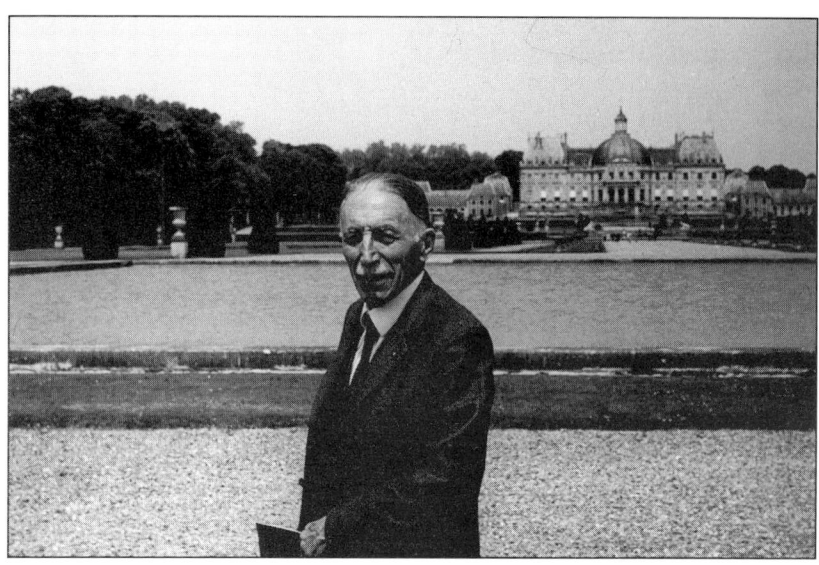
Jacques Forestier. (Eric Bywaters)

Van Breemen fought the idea that rheumatology was so wide it could not be looked upon as a system for study and that those who considered it as such were cranks—a view still held in this country in the 1930s, and by some academics as late as the early 1950s.

Ralph Pemberton could be considered as the father of American rheumatology. He was the first American physician to call himself a rheumatologist and the first American President of La Ligue Contre le Rhumatism. He became interested in arthritic problems in soldiers in World War I and established his first rheumatology clinic at the Presbyterian Hospital, Pennsylvania in 1926. He became the first Chairman of the Committee for the Study and Control of Rheumatism (CSCR) that same year and the President of its successor, the American Rheumatism Association (ARA) in 1938.

Subsequent leagues against rheumatism
The early days of La Ligue before the war were followed by the foundation of the International League and several continental and national leagues at the first post-war meeting of La Ligue at Copenhagen in 1948.

Copenhagen was a happy re-union, but Professor Pletney of Moscow surprised his friends by his outspoken criticism of some of the actions of the Soviet Union. Shortly afterwards we heard he was in prison where he died.

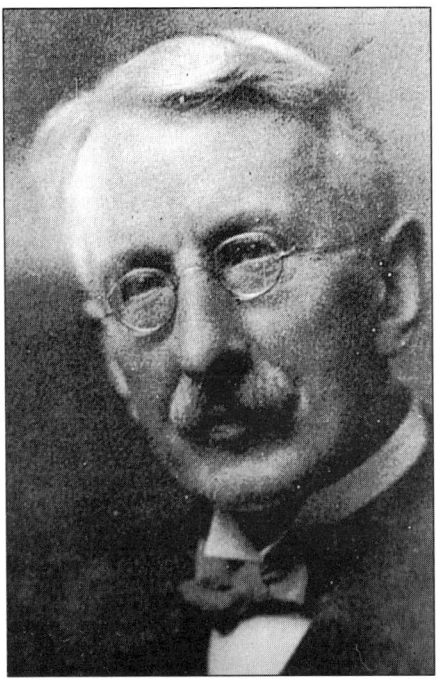

Fortescue Fox. (Eric Bywaters)

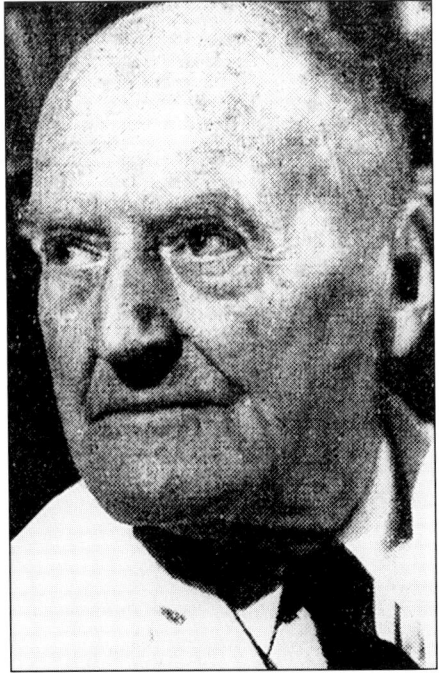

J Van Breemen. (Eric Bywaters)

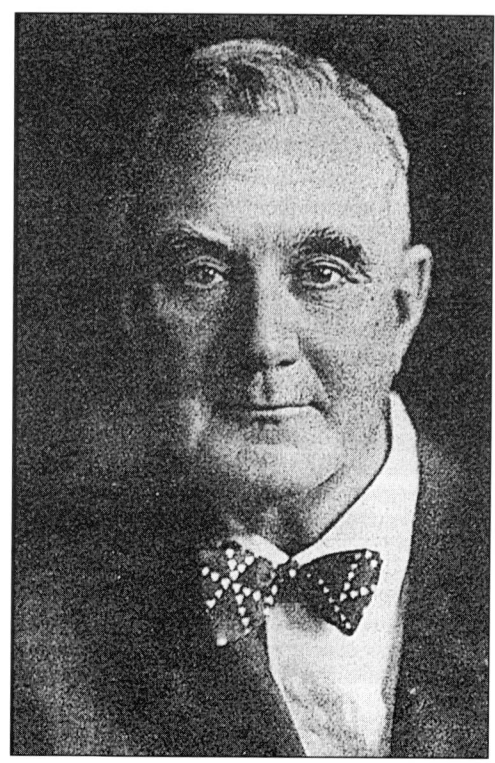

Ralph Pemberton.

The International League ILAR
The first International League Meeting was held in New York in 1949, an exciting time at the beginning of the cortisone era. The first night we arrived we had a great celebration to honour Hench, Kendall, Slocumb and Polley, the Mayo Clinic team who had made the discovery, and for which Hench and Kendall received a Nobel Prize. Ralph Pemberton was President, with Richard Freyberg, President of the American Rheumatism Association (ARA) also taking a leading part.

The Continental Leagues
The Pan American League (PANLAR) was formed in 1944 with Ralph Pemberton as President. The first European League (EULAR) meeting was held in Barcelona in 1951—Will Copeman was President. The South East Asian Pacific and Australasian League (SEAPAL) came into being in 1963 with Selwyn Nelson as President.

In EULAR a great deal of the formative work fell on the shoulders of the Secretary General, first Edstrom (Sweden), then Michotte (Belgium), Jung, (Switzerland) and Dixon (England).

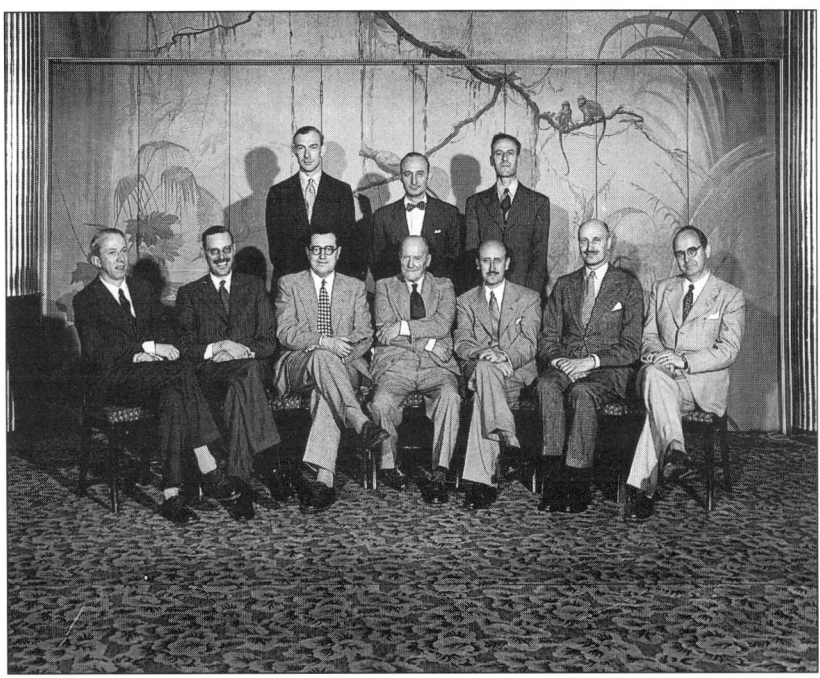

Honorary Members of the American Rheumatism Association elected to celebrate the first meeting of the International League held in New York, 1949. Honorary Members of the American Rheumatism Association, 1949.
H Burt, RH Freyberg, GD Kersley
DH Collins, W Tegner, P Barcelo, J Van Breemen, A Mareno, WSC Coptman, G Edstrom.

In the mid 1960s, with a growth in the importance of the leagues and the number of doctors attending Congresses approaching two thousand, a re-look at the structure, function and management became necessary. A federal structure of the national, continental and international leagues was agreed. Several specialised standing committees were set up to deal with education, nomenclature, epidemiology, surgery, pathology, paediatrics, drug trials and drug toxicity. A *Bulletin* to disseminate information was organised. Participation in WHO was established and prizes for research were instituted. Most important of all, a section for social agencies was formed. This was to bring in those interested or involved in rheumatology, but who were not doctors and, under the chairmanship of de Blecourt of Holland, it has had a widespread and beneficial effect on the whole organisation since its formation in 1975. In 1977 EULAR organised A World Rheumatism Year to publicise the importance of arthritis medically, socially and economically; many countries, but not the UK, produced special celebratory stamps.

My term of office (GDK) as President of EULAR gave me the opportunity of visiting many countries. What however remains most

Meeting in New York at which the International League Against Rheumatism was formed, 1949.

clearly in my mind was my visit to East Germany. Having a full programme I was at first not too keen to accept their invitation, but in retrospect I would not have missed it for anything. Usually the amount of hospitality extended to me overseas was almost embarrassing, but the doctors in the Democratic Republic, though far from wealthy, excelled with their care and welcome. They were

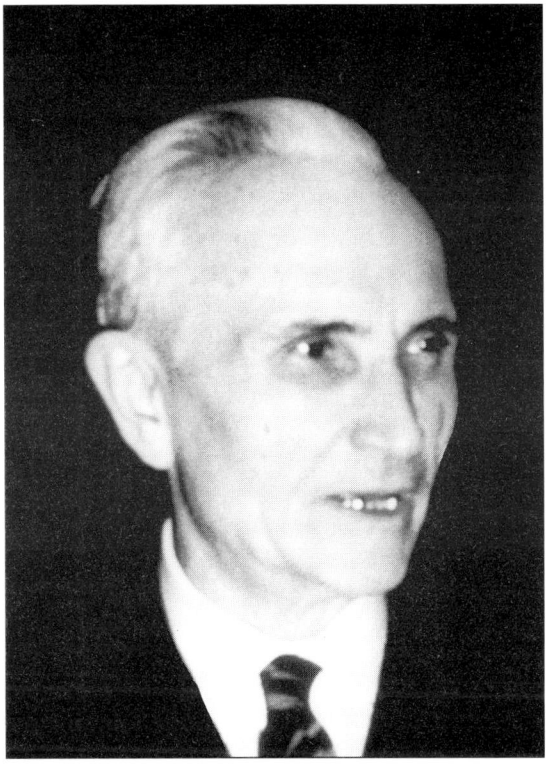
Professor Nesterov. (Eric Bywaters)

most anxious to learn all they could about what was going on in the rest of Europe and in our research projects. There were no problems so long as one kept to the letter of the law, as was evident when I was on my return journey. On arrival I had been given a few East German Deutschmarks for pocket money, but I was so well looked after that I had no chance to spend anything. After having my passport stamped at 'Checkpoint Charlie', I presented my money, and as I had no work permit, there was pandemonium, especially when I showed them my official letter of invitation to the country. They could not change the money, accept it or let me take it through the Customs. They were very apologetic, but there were no rules to cover the problem. Suddenly they had a brilliant idea—I could be marched back across the frontier, under armed guard, to spend the money—and that proved the solution.

The British League
The British League was formed in 1946, with the Officers consisting of Will Copeman, Oswald Savage and myself (GDK). It was necessary to form a British Branch in addition to the Heberden Society, as the latter had a very restricted membership and, unless an individual

was a member of the National Society which subscribed to the European League, they were debarred from attending Congresses. In 1965 to simplify matters the British League adopted the same Secretariat and Executive Committee as the Heberden Society. Then anticipating the institution of a Social Agencies Branch of EULAR, in 1972 a British counterpart BLAR, the British League Against Rheumatism, was formed. This consisted of a Scientific Section, encompassing specialists in many disciplines in addition to rheumatologists, orthopaedists, rehabilitation experts and scientists through the Heberden Society. It included also the British Association of Physical Medicine, the Back Pain Society and the British Association of Manipulative Medicine. A Social Agencies Section was also formed to include such partly lay bodies as the Arthritis and Rheumatism Council (ARC), British Rheumatism and Arthritis Association (BRAA), the British Council for Rehabilitation of the Disabled (BCRD), the Back Pain Association (BPA) and the Horder Homes. Dr Michael Mason was elected President, with Dr AC Boyle, Chairman of the Scientific Section and Lord Tweedsmuir Chairman of the Social Agencies Section. Michael Mason was followed as President by Colin Barnes and then Professor Maini.

Jacques Forestier seemed to embody the spirit of La Ligue Contre Le Rhumatism, always ready to help with any problem. Professor Nesterov of Moscow for many years headed the contingent from behind the 'iron curtain'. The Russian party, usually of four including the interpreter, appeared at first very daunting never mixing with the remainder, till at last one really got to know Nesterov. He then became human and humorous, but still pretended to speak only Russian, until one day in his excitement he broke into voluble and excellent French.

Early physiotherapy
At the beginning of this century a scientific interest in physical therapy was developing with the work by Winternitz in Vienna, Di Caspero in Graz, Von Leyden in Berlin, Baruch in New York, Finsen working on ultra violet radiation and Van Breemen in Amsterdam.

Apart from at the spas, it was in the 1920s that departments of physiotherapy started up in the London teaching hospitals. Sir Robert Stanton Woods established a Department of Physical Medicine at the London Hospital in 1921 and shortly afterwards Cumberbatch did so at St Bartholomew's Hospital. Sir Morton Smart had a large Harley Street practice using various light rays. Most treatments consisted of radiant heat and massage with prostatic diathermy and sometimes the use of terrifying shocks from a Wimshurst machine to break down adhesions. Nearly all treatment was passive, though in Sweden exercises were coming into vogue. At St Thomas's Hospital, JB Mennell was teaching the elements of manipulation, concentrating on traction and then freeing up movements not under voluntary control.

Most manipulations were, however, carried out by the non-medically qualified bone setters such as Barker. In those days litigation hardly existed and little was heard about the subsequent disasters.

Chapter 2

The 1930s

It was in the 1930s that rheumatology as we know it first saw the light of day though it was Alison Glover's *Reports on the Incidence of the Rheumatic Diseases (1924-28)* that did much to provoke official interest, and prompted the Royal College of Physicians to form a Committee on their nomenclature and classification.

The clinical picture
What was the clinical picture at that time?

In 1932, the teaching of rheumatology at St Bartholomew's Hospital consisted at most of two short talks by an orthopaedic surgeon and, if a rheumatoid patient was admitted, probably because she had been seen privately by a consultant, she was sandwiched between a patient with haematemesis and one with diabetic coma and was passed over on the ward round. Outside hospitals one saw 'Grannie', who had been in the attic for many years, with knees under her chin and with fingers so flexed that the nails had grown into and through her hand. Spondylitics were so bent that, standing, they could see only the ground and sometimes it was easier to progress backwards, looking between their legs than trying to see in front of them.

Yet whole wards were full of cases of rheumatic fever and whole hospitals with bone and joint tuberculosis. Treatment depended on the doctor rather than on the disease. It often consisted of elimination of imaginary sepsis in teeth, tonsils, sinuses, gall bladder, appendix, or of colonic lavage to remove noxious bacteria. It was thought that all rheumatism must be caused by an infection and must be eradicated or alternatively that an autogenous vaccine should be used.

Later gold was used in controlled dosage, often causing exfoliative dermatitis and renal damage. Dosage was too high, early signs of toxicity were not recognised and there was no consensus of opinion whether to continue treatment for life or to use the short, sharp shock method. Other treatments used were protein shock, with disastrous effects, and electric shocks from the terrifying Wimshurst machine. Hydrotherapy plus aspirin was the best any 'rheumatic' could hope for, though of course haematemesis was a common result. Complete surgical excision of the head and neck of the femur was the most effective orthopaedic help and this, after a lengthy and painful convalescence, left the patient with a most unstable gait.

In ankylosing spondylitis, considered a type of rheumatoid arthritis, radiotherapy was used with considerable benefit as a routine, both locally, to the whole spine, or as a general irradiation. Then came the knowledge of the risk of provoking leukaemia. Rest in a plaster bed for months to try and prevent deformity was the rule, rather than the mobilisation practised today, and this resulted in completely stiff backs.

In gout, amputation of tophaceous toes and fingers was often a necessity. Colchicine was pushed until it produced diarrhoea and vomiting to control attacks, together with cinchophen as a longer term uric acid eliminator and this, from time to time, caused acute yellow atrophy of the liver and death. After 1927, salicylates were used in large dosages as uricosurics, clogging the kidneys with uric acid crystals.

Since then there has been a complete revolution in the treatment of arthritis and the rheumatic diseases, as well as in the attitude of the medical profession. It is therefore of interest to review some of the landmarks. To begin with, there has been a virtual disappearance of rheumatic fever and tuberculosis of bone and joints, except in the Third World, and satisfactory control of gout. The polymyalgia rheumatica syndrome was described by George Kersley at the League meeting in Spain in 1951 as 'a myalgic syndrome of the aged with systemic reaction and responding to cortisone'; it had often been confused with carcinomatosis. The connective tissue diseases have been recognised and, perhaps of most clinical significance, have been the advances of surgery into the treatment of arthritis.

Rheumatic fever, first described by Wells in 1812[1] and Bouillaud in 1886,[2] with its cardiac pathology defined by Aschoff in 1904,[3] was the first rheumatic condition to be eliminated. Starting with Lancefield's discovery of the significance of the *Streptococcus viridans* in 1940[4] there followed the use of antibiotics and better hygiene.

Gout, first pathologically distinguished by Garrod in 1848,[5] became partly controlled by the uricosurics with the work of Jennings on salicylates in 1927,[6] by the use of Benemid by Talbott in 1951[7] and then the breakthrough with the discovery of the genetically determined xanthine oxidase inhibition by Rundles[8] and then Seegmiller.[9] Uric acid production then became controlled, instead of only its excess being partly eliminated, often at the expense of renal problems. This step forward was followed by the discovery of the crystal induced arthritides, starting with the demonstration of calcium pyro-phosphate in chondrocalcinosis by McCarty of Wisconsin[10] and Sitaj of Piestany[11] and apatite deposition by Dieppe.[12]

Interest in the 'connective tissue diseases' can be attributed to Hench, Kendall, Slocumb and Polley's work on the anti-inflammatory effect of the steroids[13] and Hans Selye's concept of stress on the immunological system.[14] But before this, the work of

Klemperer and Baehr on connective tissue did much to stimulate research in this field.[15]

Some understanding of the immunogenetics and now the molecular biology of these diseases dates back to Waaler of Oslo's agglutination of sensitised sheep's red cells by certain sera in 1937[16] and Rose *et al* of the USA showing its relationship to rheumatoid arthritis in 1948.[17] Also in 1948 Hargraves described the LE cell, blazing the way to the study of auto-antibodies to nuclear antigens.[18] Then in 1964 Lilly reported viral and genetic factors causing leukemogenesis in certain strains of mice.[19] All this work has contributed to the present day treatment by immunosuppressive drugs and has opened up areas of research into the causation and future therapy of connective tissue disease.

Finally the recognition of the importance of osteoporosis in postmenopausal women has led to investigation and demonstration of the value of mobility and hormonal treatment in this widespread and disabling condition.

Yet even today, despite the numerous non-steroidal anti-inflammatory drugs and disease modifying anti-rheumatic agents, their very number indicates that none are wholly satisfactory. Even combined with immunosuppression, we have no cure for rheumatoid arthritis. The gross deformities are now prevented and more comfort is obtained. Working life can also be prolonged. But this is as far as we have progressed, despite the concentration of some of the best brains in the country on the problem. Perhaps this scientific interest is the greatest and most hopeful change over the last 60 years.

Orthopaedics
The surgical treatment of the rheumatic diseases, both of soft tissue and bone, has been one of the greatest recent steps forward from the purely therapeutic point of view. Ortho-paedia, meaning 'straight child', was originally almost confined to the treatment of children with tuberculosis, osteomyelitis and the after effects of poliomyelitis. Though the British Orthopaedic Society was founded in 1894, it was World War I which put orthopaedics, as we know it today, on the map. It was not, however, till 1918 that the British Orthopaedic Association was formed, shortly after its American counterpart, and largely due to the input of Sir Robert Jones and the American Surgeon Robert Osgood. There are now over 700 members.

The progress in orthopaedics is best exemplified by hip arthroplasty. It started as the pre-World War II Girdlestone excision, a painful procedure often leading to instability and mainly used for the worst spondylitics. Then followed the Smith-Peterson vitallium cup.[20] In 1946 the Judet acrylic head followed[21] and in 1952 the Moore vitallium ball and socket.[22] In 1960 came the real breakthrough by John Charnley[23] with his low friction small

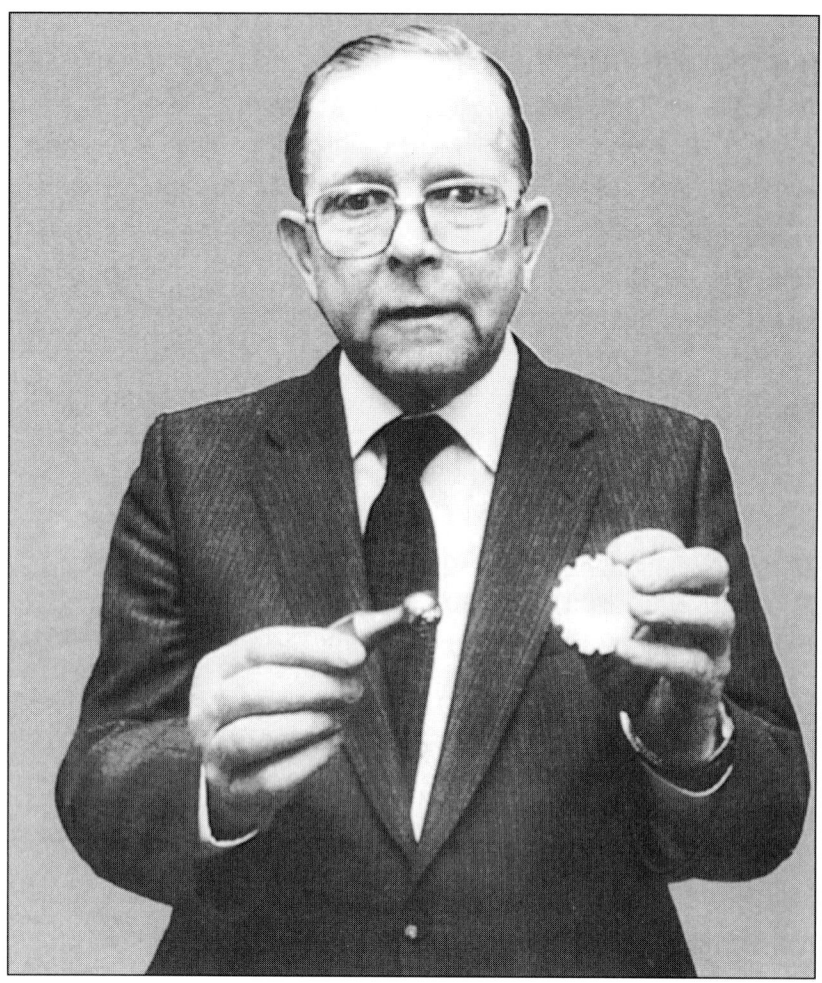

Sir John Charnley.

vitallium metal head and high density polyethylene plastic socket fixed with cement, which did much to reduce tissue reactions and increase stability. He then tackled the other great problem of infection with a 'theatre within the theatre' and more regular preventive use of antibiotics. Now 50,000 total hip replacements are performed annually in Britain alone with an overall 80% ten-year success rate. Following on the success in hip surgery, in 1970 Michael Freeman produced the condylar knee prosthesis with capping of the bone ends rather than removal of a large quantity of bone, thus reducing the trauma and increasing efficiency of the operation. Many other joints now are being successfully replaced and soft tissue surgery and tendon replants are becoming commonplace.

Teaching has improved dramatically. Even in the late 1940s Birmingham was considered progressive when Professor Wilkinson sent his final year students to Bath for one day's clinical instruction, an example followed in a couple of years by Bristol.

One aspect of rheumatology in which there has, however, been little progress in knowledge or treatment has been in fibrositis or fibromyalgia as it is now known.

In 1816 Scudamore first described the most widespread and to this day most neglected rheumatic syndrome named by Sir William Gowers in 1902 and then Stockman in 1920 'fibrositis'. The latter found inflammatory changes around the connective tissue involved in skeletal muscles and tendons. This was not substantiated subsequently and the term became a dirty word and the syndrome a 'waste paper basket' for the lazy or incompetent to dump cases they could not place in any other recognised category.

The condition consisted of pain and tenderness in the muscles, especially common in the neck and shoulders, often with what appears to be tender nodules, disappearing under anaesthesia. They are common in tense and pain sensitive individuals, most frequently women, exacerbated by local chilling, trauma, infections and fatigue. Localised muscle and vascular spasm may play a part. It used to be common in those who had previously had rheumatic fever and was exacerbated by 'weather fronts', which especially in ectomorphs can produce vasoconstriction and some tissue hypoxia. This is particularly the case in areas of abnormal scar tissue.

Recently the attitude of the medical profession to this neglected syndrome has begun to change and to make a break with its disreputable past reputation the condition has been re-named fibromyalgia, which also ceases to presuppose the inflammatory nature of the condition and links it with irritability of the bowel, headaches and anxiety, but still there is no adequate therapy. Normal management involves reassurance that the pain is real but not 'dangerous', and administration of analgesics during exacerbations. Heat, massage, exercises and relaxation are helpful.

It is hoped that more research into this condition, which many rheumatologists think affects 50% of their patients, will be now forthcoming. In eleven out of fifteen biopsies of tender areas in the trapezius muscles, focal loss of a specific enzyme and 'moth eaten' fibres were found. Electronmicroscopy of five specimens revealed mitochondrial abnormalities in all cases. These findings could be due to increases in muscle tension.[24]

The beginning of rheumatology

It was just after I (GDK) had been successful in the Membership Examination in 1933 that I suddenly realised that, though I could have answered a question on some brain tumour that I might never see, I would have felt a question on rheumatoid arthritis unfair. I was then Chief Assistant, today equivalent to Senior Registrar, on the Medical Unit at St Bartholomew's Hospital, so I consulted my 'chief', Professor Sir Frances Fraser. The reaction was dramatic. He told me I would be prostituting my soul if I 'left Barts to associate with all the quacks of the Universe'. I replied that if that was the attitude, how could medicine improve? His response to this was most generous and he promised to help me all he could. He recommended me for appointment to the Royal College's Committee and wrote the preface to my first book.

I then had the temerity to visit Sir Wilson Jamieson, the Chief Medical Officer of Health, and ask him why no governmental effort was being put into the treatment of the rheumatic diseases. His reply I never forgot—'I agree with you. Now go out and stimulate public opinion to make me do more.'

Sir Thomas, later Lord Horder, who had been my other chief at St Bartholomew's Hospital, was the one person who gave me, from the first, enthusiastic encouragement and who later became a personal friend.

Fraser and Horder, though both great men, could not have been more different. Fraser was the academic, with knowledge of all the most recent literature and, when preparing a difficult case for consultation, he would go into the pros and cons of every possibility before calling Horder in. 'Tommy' would sit on or by the patient's bed, holding his or her hand, ask a few questions, carry out what appeared to be a cursory examination, immediately pronounce the diagnosis, and was *never* wrong. He used to say diagnosis is easy but prognosis less certain. It was this diagnostic sixth sense that put him at the top of his profession against all the odds.

Lord Horder was born in 1871. He started at St Bartholomew's Hospital with no money, virtually disinherited by his father because he would not go into the family drapery business in Shaftesbury. Though most thoughtful of his juniors, he had a waspish tongue when challenged by his seniors and delighted in showing up their inefficiencies and mistakes. He must have been unpopular with many seniors, but his clinical brilliance was irrepressible. He was again always willing to defend what at the time were unpopular causes if he felt they were worthwhile, whether it was cremation, noise abatement or the spas. I well remember, at a dinner of the British Spas Federation of which he was President, how he reduced to pulp a senior professor, who had attended as a guest, and then denigrated the spas. His vital backing of causes, at the time unaccepted, did not provoke popularity with some of the academics. It was however his initiative in the fight to promote rheumatology and later rehabilitation as orthodox specialties that was of outstanding importance and which did so much to advance by a number of years the time of their acceptance. He was the first Chairman of the ERC, a President of the Heberden Society and the first President of the BAPM. He did not just give his name to these

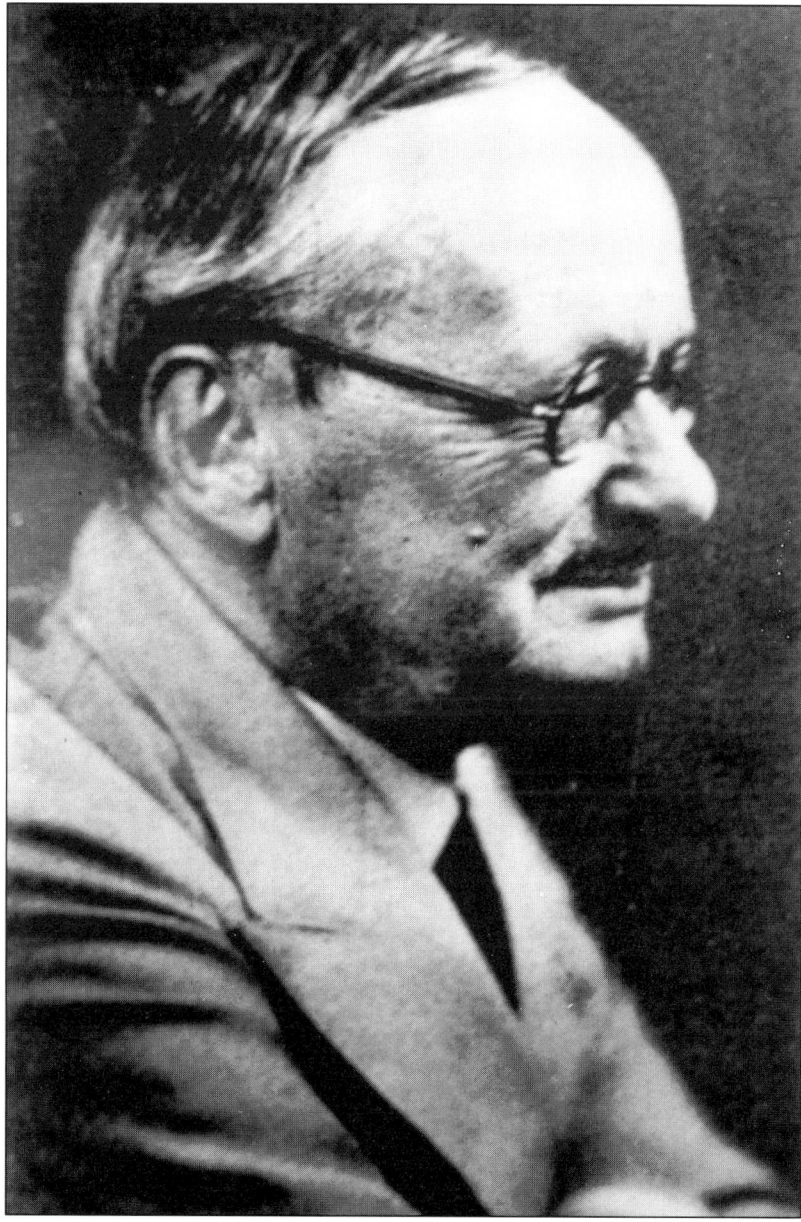

Lord Horder. (Eric Bywaters)

organisations, but worked hard to get them established. Till the end he was full of energy. A year before he died in 1955 at the age of 84, he left Petersfield, gave a broadcast interview in London on obesity, came down to Bath for a party and dinner of the Fellowship for Freedom in Medicine and apologised for leaving early next morning to organise some work in his garden.

With Horder's backing I decided to leave St Bartholomew's Hospital and return to my birth place, Bath, to continue medicine with rheumatology as my specialty, thus following in the steps of Will Copeman, the first physician to take up the challenge.

Will Copeman, born in 1900, trained at St Thomas's Hospital, started in paediatrics and then made the field of rheumatology his main objective in life, guiding it into respectability. The Middlesex Hospital and Peto Place in London were his first footholds

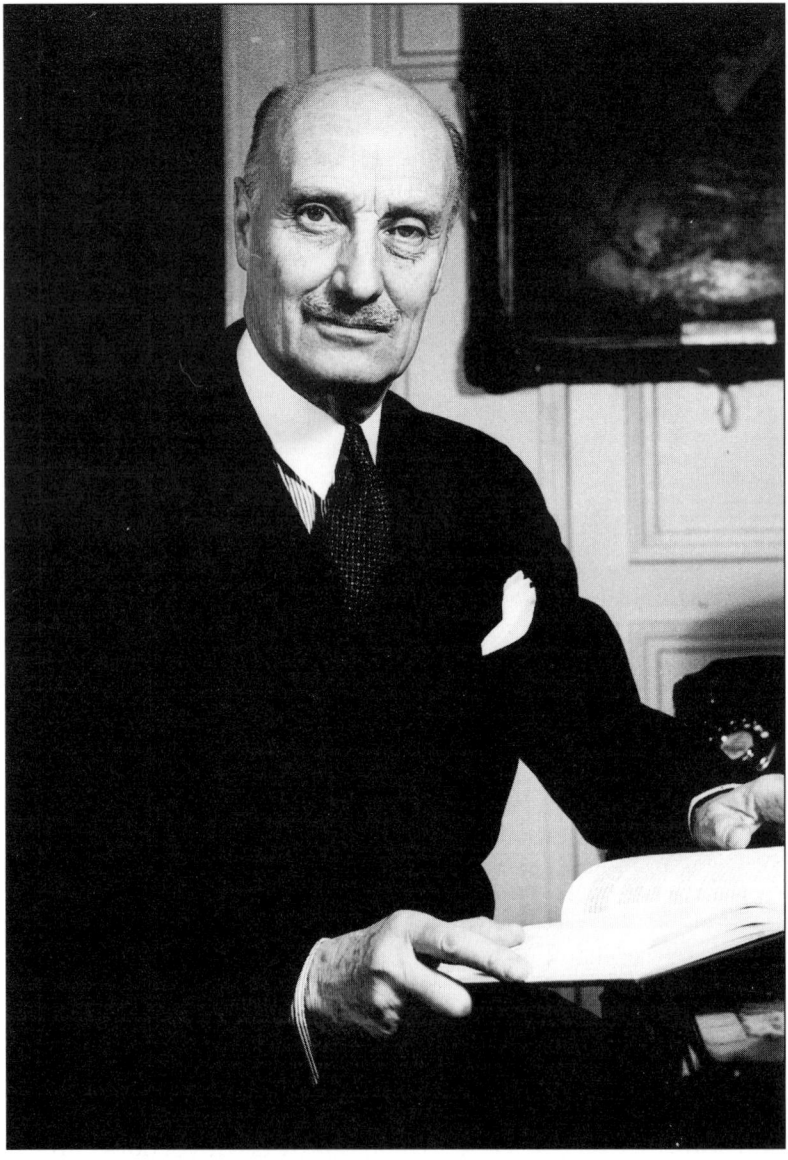

Will Copeman. (Elizabeth Dawson)

in this battle. He was the first Medical Secretary and later Chairman of the ERC and became a Heberden President and Orator.

He and I took our MDs at Cambridge together, though he was six years my senior. We were friends ever after. He was I think a little disgusted at my temporarily going into physical medicine as part of the war effort. He always fought for rheumatology to remain as a respectable specialty of internal medicine and against any link up with rehabilitation. He was also against co-operation between the ERC and the lay British Rheumatism Association, headed by Francis Bach. Copeman's objective was to prevent academic rheumatology, in the guise of the ERC and Heberden Society, from being contaminated by more dubious organisations. He was not at all enthusiastic when Horder and I joined the BRA (now Arthritis Care). Horder and I alone thought the two organisations should work in parallel rather than in competition. In all his battles he was most ably assisted and guided by his wife, Helen. Despite his serious and very respectable side, he could relax and become very human. With Horder's support and guidance he did more than anyone to put British rheumatology on its feet. He died in 1970.

When I decided to make a break with St Bartholomew's Hospital to study rheumatology, I hoped also to continue with internal medicine, and Bath was the obvious choice. Here was the Royal Mineral Water Hospital (the Min), ripe for development for rheumatological treatment, research and teaching. In addition there was also an excellent general hospital, the Royal United (RUH). I was lucky, despite my youth, in obtaining an honorary appointment as Consultant to both.

The RUH was perhaps the best non-teaching general hospital in this country, with more Fellows of the Royal College of Physicians on its staff than its bigger teaching rival at Bristol. There was also a small eye hospital and an ENT hospital. The RUH had recently moved out from the centre of Bath to a new prestigious building. As a Cambridge student I had worked in the vacations in the old hospital, assisting the surgeons, often also GPs, with their operations. They preferred my young agile hands to those of another often elderly GP.

The Min was in the building opened in 1742 and in another built in the same style in 1861. It had been little altered since, was dark and, with segregation of the sexes, even the bridge joining the two buildings was separated so that the women and men would never meet. It was staffed by an elderly Resident Medical Officer who resisted change and it was visited by consultants, who in some cases were mainly interested in the RUH, but wished to have their names on the board and to carry out some spa private practice.

The hospital was controlled by a Board of Governors consisting of elderly benefactors, many retired Admirals and Generals and the medical staff who were of course honorary. They left routine matters to a Committee, on which I immediately found myself, and where most of the remainder were old enough to be my father. Vincent Coates and myself and our great benefactor Sidney Robinson were the only ones who really wanted a change to modernise the antiquity of the institution.

Any aspiring young consultant bought a house in the Circus, the 'pill box', where he lived with his family and practised from the ground floor. Unpaid for his hospital work, he did general practice and gradually reduced this if the handling of his hospital work brought in private consultations.

But things were moving. Vincent Coates, my immediate senior, was in his early forties and had his Fellowship; he also was a rugger cap. He was keen for a change and our first job was to remove the Resident Medical Officer and to bring in younger juniors. Unfortunately not long after this Vincent Coates walked out of a moving train on the way back from a rugger dinner and was found dead on the line.

A Governor, Sidney Robinson, gave the hospital a great deal of money and also paid for a whole time research worker, Walter Leventhal. He had an animal house built and then started to carry out some of the first work on immunological factors in rheumatoid arthritis. His work was published in the early part of World War II and its significance was little recognised. In this pre-war period Leslie Hill and Barnes Burt both joined us from Buxton, and Charles Kindersley, a surgeon, was one of the first to institute plaster treatment and manipulation for arthritic deformities.

Plans were started to build a new hospital and this was only halted by the war, which was declared eight days before the Queen was to lay its foundation stone. By that time, in 1936, we had changed the name of the hospital, by Act of Parliament, to the Royal National Hospital for Rheumatic Diseases to signify that we now treated arthritis by every method known to us, rather than attempt to wash away gallstones with the mineral water. It was the first spa hospital to move into the era of super scientific reaction to quackery. With the swing of the pendulum anything that could not be proven did not exist, thus completely ignoring the effect of the psyche and our present day more holistic approach.

In those days most cases of rheumatic disease were referred to the orthopaedists, and there were few of these outside the major teaching hospitals. As late as 1948, when I was appointed Regional Advisor in Rheumatology, Norman Capener, a personal friend and the uncrowned king of orthopaedics in the West, told me there was no need for my help with rheumatic cases in his domain, except to advise as to whether their hearts were in a fit condition for him to operate. Yet in Bath we have the famous 1742 painting by Hoare showing a consultation between Dr Oliver and Jeremy Peirce the surgeon, almost 200 years before such co-operation became generally acceptable (page 2).

Participants in the beginning of rheumatology in the UK

The Royal College of Physicians
This august body has played an important, if unsung role in the history of rheumatology. Firstly it was the forerunner of the ERC, then during the chaotic period of the early 1950s it helped to sort out the problems of the specialty and its interrelationship with physical medicine, orthopaedics and general medicine. Even today it is stressing the inadequacy of clinical cover in rheumatology in many parts of the country.

Stimulated by the *Reports on Rheumatic Diseases* of Dr Alison Glover of the Ministry of Health in 1924-28, the College in 1932 set up a committee to study the classification and nomenclature of the rheumatic diseases under the chairmanship of Sir Humphrey Rolleston with such notabilities as Lord Horder, Sir Francis Fraser, Sir William Willcox, Dr Alison Glover and Dr Fortescue Fox and with Sir Robert Hutchinson, as President of the College ex-officio. Will Copeman was Secretary, Charles Buckley Editor of the *Reports* and Alan Moncrieff represented paediatrics. It was this committee that was the forerunner of the ERC and published the *Reports on Rheumatic Diseases*; which eventually became the *Annals of the Rheumatic Diseases*.

After World War II, The College in 1948 instituted the Diploma of Physical Medicine. In 1950 it set up a Rheumatology Committee, chaired by the President, which decided that the specialty of rheumatology could be entered from general medicine, orthopaedics or physical medicine. In some centres it would be a whole-time specialty combined with research and teaching. Alternatively it could be a part-time specialty within the framework of internal medicine or it could be combined with rehabilitation which would involve taking charge of physical medicine departments.

The Rt Hon Winston Churchill became an Honorary Fellow of the Royal College of Physicians in 1951 and presented a portrait to Lord Moran.

The Empire Rheumatism Council (ERC, ARC)
When the College's Rheumatology Committee of 1932 had completed its work and published its *Reports on Rheumatic Diseases*, Lord Horder and Will Copeman decided, at a meeting at the Royal Society of Medicine in 1936, to carry on the good work by founding the ERC. The Duke of Gloucester agreed to be President and Sir Theodor Fox was engaged as Secretary General. A full history of the ERC and its successor the Arthritis and Rheumatism Council (ARC) is

Empire Rheumatism Council

President:
H.R.H. THE DUKE OF GLOUCESTER, K.G.

Chairman:
Dr. W. S. C. COPEMAN, O.B.E., F.R.C.P.

Vice-Chairman:
Professor SIR CHARLES DODDS, M.V.O., F.R.C.P., F.R.S.

NATIONAL 21st BIRTHDAY
£250,000 FUND

Chairman of the Fund:
Col. THE Rt. Hon. THE LORD ASTOR OF HEVER, LL.D.

Patrons

SIR EDWARD BARON
COLONEL DENIS BATES, M.C., T.D.
WILFRED B. BEARD, ESQ., O.B.E.
H. P. BIBBY, ESQ.
The Rt. Hon. The LORD BILSLAND, K.T., M.C., D.L., LL.D.
SIR ERIC BOWATER
SIR JAMES BOWMAN, K.B.E.
J. CAMPBELL, ESQ.
W. J. CARRON, ESQ.
FRANK COUSINS, ESQ.
The Rt. Hon. The EARL OF DUDLEY, M.C., T.D., D.L.
Lt.-Col. The Rt. Hon. The LORD DUDLEY GORDON, D.S.O.
The Rt. Hon. The EARL OF ELGIN AND KINCARDINE, K.T., C.M.G., T.D.

SIR JOHN HANBURY-WILLIAMS, C.V.O.
The Rt. Hon. The LORD HEYWORTH
SIR ELLIS HUNTER
W. E. JONES, ESQ., O.B.E.
The Rt. Hon. The LORD KINDERSLEY, C.B.E., M.C.
The Rt. Hon. The VISCOUNT KNOLLYS, G.C.M.G., M.B.E. D.F.C.
SIR PERCY LISTER
SIR GEORGE NELSON, Bt.
GENERAL SIR BRIAN ROBERTSON, G.C.B., G.B.E., K.C.M.G., K.C.V.O., D.S.O., M.C.
J. P. SAVAGE, ESQ.
SIR VINCENT TEWSON, C.B.E., M.C.
SIR THOMAS WILLIAMSON, C.B.E.

FARADAY HOUSE, 8/10 CHARING CROSS ROAD,
LONDON, W.C.2

Empire Rheumatism Council, 21st Birthday Celebration, 1947. Guests at the top table.

being researched and compiled at present, so this will be only an abbreviated and anecdotal account of the most important organisation in the story of rheumatology. Few can have dreamed that this small body with a budget of a few thousand pounds, would today be dispensing annually some £10 million on research and teaching.

The heart of the organisation was the Scientific Advisory Committee, chaired by Sir William Willcox. With growth in prestige, more and more distinguished doctors were incorporated, till Horder decided it was becoming unwieldy and demoted a large number of them to less important sub-committees. Francis Bach was one of these and, unfortunately, he was much hurt and was never again such a firm supporter. In the post-war years he became the doyen of the British Rheumatic Association (BRA) and this, perhaps with some feeling that he worked in the Emergency Medical Services at home rather than largely overseas, caused the rift with Will Copeman, to whom the ERC and Heberden Society were the only respectable 'rheumatological' bodies. Francis Bach was a very kind man and adored by his patients, though he was perhaps not so academically brilliant as some. He did a great deal to steer the BRA into becoming an important organisation, which should have worked in parallel rather than in rivalry with the ERC.

Sir Theodor Fox was succeeded as Secretary General of the ERC by Victor Howell and then by Michael Andrews. The latter, though a quiet, unassuming man, did more than anyone to steer the ARC into its present secure financial position. He guided the officers, often I think without them realising it, into a wise course.

In 1964, having budded off the Canadian, New Zealand and Australian Councils, the ERC changed its name to the ARC. It is now flourishing under the Patronage of the Duchess of Kent with Lord Porritt as President and Colin Barnes has taken over the Chairmanship from the late Michael Mason. It would be impossible to list all that the Council has achieved, but it was actively involved in the formation of the Chairs of Rheumatology at Manchester in 1958 and later at the London Postgraduate Hospital, Edinburgh, Glasgow, the London Hospital, Leeds and Bristol (see Appendix for dates and holders).

The ARC was largely responsible for the formation of the Epidemiology Unit at Manchester in 1954, the Kennedy Research Institute of Rheumatology in 1966 and the Bone and Joint Unit at the London Hospital in 1974. It also organised an extension of the Rheumatology Departments at the Royal Northern Hospital in Edinburgh, of the Middlesex Hospital and the Bio-Engineering Unit at Leeds. It has sponsored in the past industrial, drug and electronmicroscopy units. It has founded many Lectureships and Research Fellowships and makes block grants to 19 hospitals in addition to individual research grants. It provided headquarters and general secretariat for the Heberden Society with which it was affiliated.

The ARC has now in 1989 broken the barrier of the £10 million mark raised in one year for research and teaching, has over 1200 branches and supports six Professorial Chairs. Lord Arthur Porritt, a great friend of Will Copeman's since their early years at

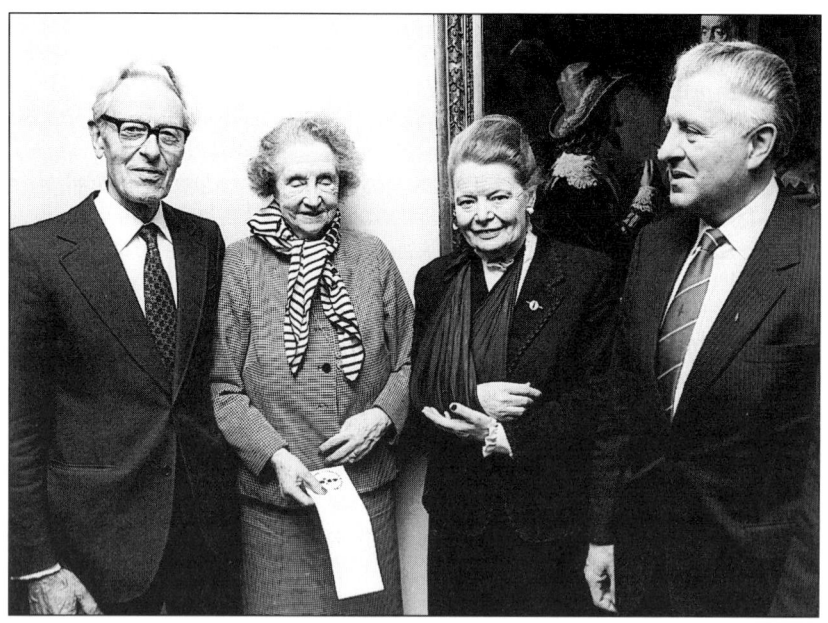

All Branches meeting of ARC.
George Kersley, Mrs Pryor (Bath representative), Rt Hon Hornsby-Smith (Vice-Chairman ARC), Colin G Barnes (Chairman ARC Scientific Committee), 1985.

Cambridge, has recently, after twelve years as President, handed over this office to Lord Dainton.

Peto Place and the Arthur Stanley Institute
The two reputable organisations that gave birth to rheumatology in the 1930s were the ERC, dealing with fund raising for research and teaching, and its clinical complement the Heberden Society. The latter evolved from the Staff Committee of the Peto Place Red Cross Clinic, where most of the reputable London physicians interested in rheumatic diseases worked and where, after World War II, even 'Pat' Patterson and myself came up from Droitwich and Bath to do clinics on alternate weeks.

It was in 1930 that the Red Cross Clinic at Peto Place was opened by Queen Mary for the treatment of rheumatic disease, largely by hydro- and physio-therapy. Queen Mary became President; His Majesty the King was patron and the Duke of Gloucester was Chairman of Council. One floor of the building was reserved for private patients and the remainder for those less well off and treated for a reduced fee. There was also a Samaritan fund to pay for those who could afford nothing. Sir Arthur Stanley was the Chairman and Matthew Ray, Frank Howitt, CB Heald, JS Nissen and WSC Copeman were the medical consultants.

With the arrival of the NHS this clinic became affiliated to the Middlesex Hospital and became the Arthur Stanley Institute; in 1965 it was amalgamated with the Middlesex Hospital and moved to new purpose-built accommodation as its Physical Medicine Department.

It was at Peto Place, Bath and Buxton that schools for training in hydrotherapy were started and achieved recognition by the Chartered Society of Physiotherapists.

The Heberden Society
Although the Heberden Society was the clinical and research breakthrough of the 1930s, its history will only be summarised. For detail and full biographies of all its Presidents, Orators and Roundsmen reference may be made to Moll's major work *The Heberden Society* 1987, which deals exclusively with this subject.

The Heberden Society was founded in 1936 as a clinical and scientific society for the advancement of the study of the rheumatic diseases by six physicians on the staff of the aforementioned British Red Cross Society's Clinic for Rheumatism at Peto Place, then under the chairmanship of Dr Matthew Ray. This was then known as the Committee for the Study and Investigation of Rheumatism. A year later membership was thrown open to all medical men interested in rheumatology, up to a maximum number of 100, and the name was then changed to the Heberden Society with Frank Howitt as President. In the same year Dr CB Heald presented the Heberden medal. This is now awarded annually and was recast in its present form during the Presidency of Lord Cohen of Birkenhead. Recipients have included a number of distinguished men from overseas including the two Nobel Prize Laureates, Hench and Kendall.

The Society's valuable historical library was founded in 1938. This now comprises some 500 volumes and manuscripts and is housed for the Society in the Heberden Room at the Royal College of Physicians of London. Its development was largely due to Will Copeman and then Eric Bywaters.

The Society continued to meet regularly until 1940, when its ordinary meetings could no longer be held because of the war. During this period, however, the Committee continued to meet and the Heberden medal was awarded on two occasions.

Regular meetings were renewed when the war ended in 1945, and a new constitution, based upon that of the Association of Physicians of Great Britain and Ireland was adopted.

The *Annals of the Rheumatic Diseases* became the official organ of the society, which affiliated itself to the ERC (now the Arthritis and Rheumatism Council for Research) towards the end of that year. Three years later the Annual Heberden Round was instituted and was first conducted by the then Regius Professor of Physic in Cambridge,

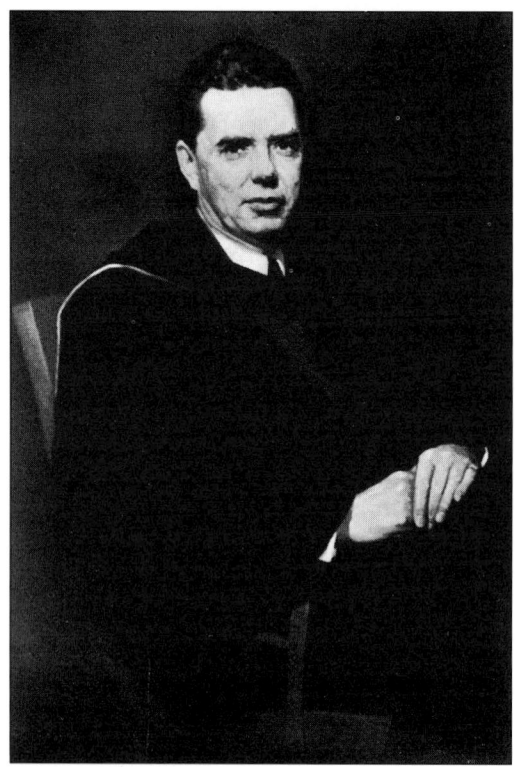

Phillip Hench.

Sir Lionel Whitby. This was followed by a dinner in Heberden's college, St John's, at which the Vice-Chancellor presided. The annual dinner then became an event attended by many distinguished guests, amongst whom may be mentioned the Princess Royal, the Duchess of Kent, several Ministers of Health, a Lord Chancellor, a Lord Privy Seal, and the Reverend Edward Heberden, a surviving descendant of William Heberden. The Presidents of both senior Royal Colleges accepted membership ex-officio under the new constitution. By 1951, the pressure to join the Society had become such that the new categories of Associate, and in 1954 Overseas Membership, were instituted. In 1972 the Constitution was revised to enlarge its membership and give voting rights to Associate Members.

It is not recorded why William Heberden, MD, FRCP, FRS (1710-1801) was selected as our 'father of rheumatology'. His more important medical work was on angina and chickenpox rather than on the finger nodes for which he is best known. He was however a great scholar and highly religious. One wonders if Will Copeman, also an erudite medical historian, suggested his name in deference to his literary achievements.

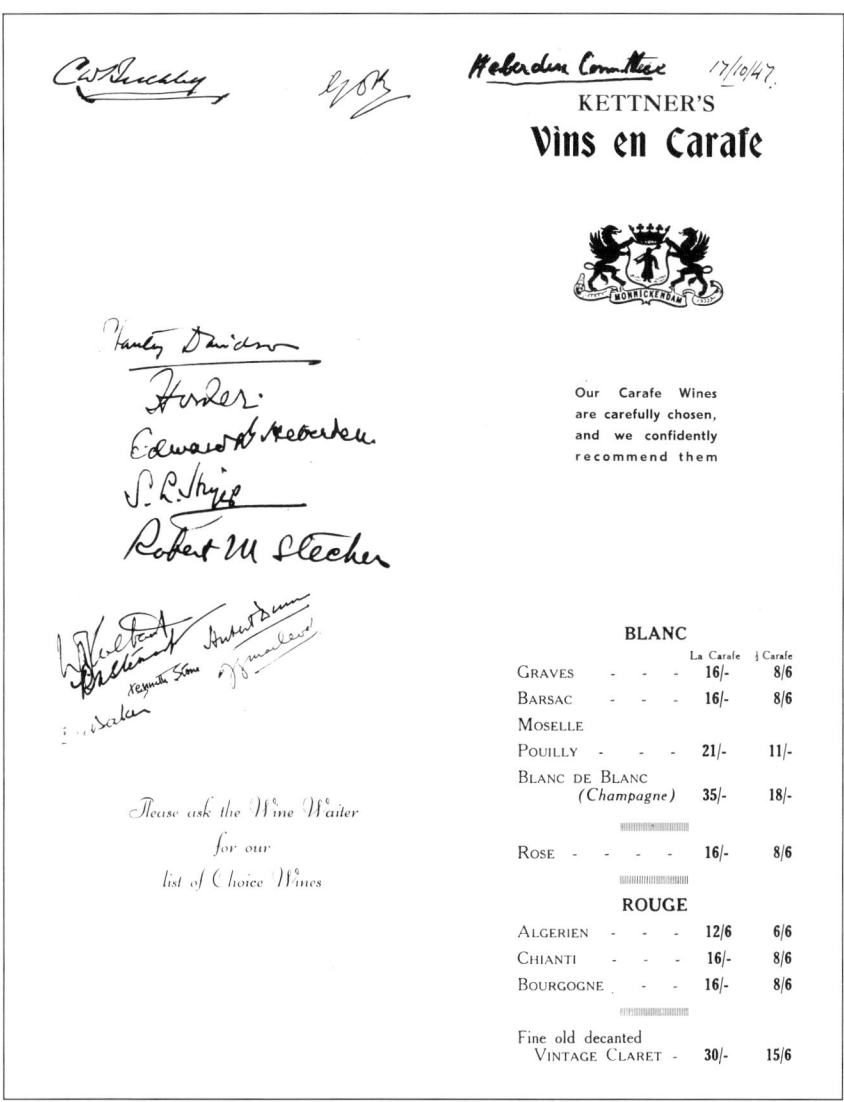

Wine list signed by committee members of the Heberden Society, 1947.

The names and dates of the Presidents, Roundsmen and Orators will be found in the Appendix and among them are many of the important physicians of this decade. Will Copeman became the first post-war President followed by Henry Cohen, later Lord Cohen, and then in 1953 by Lord Horder.

It is interesting how Cohen became involved. He was a brilliant man with a photographic memory—as a student he could recite most of Price's textbook of medicine word for word. He was President of the British Medical Association, of the General Medical Council, of the Royal Society of Medicine and of the Association of Physicians

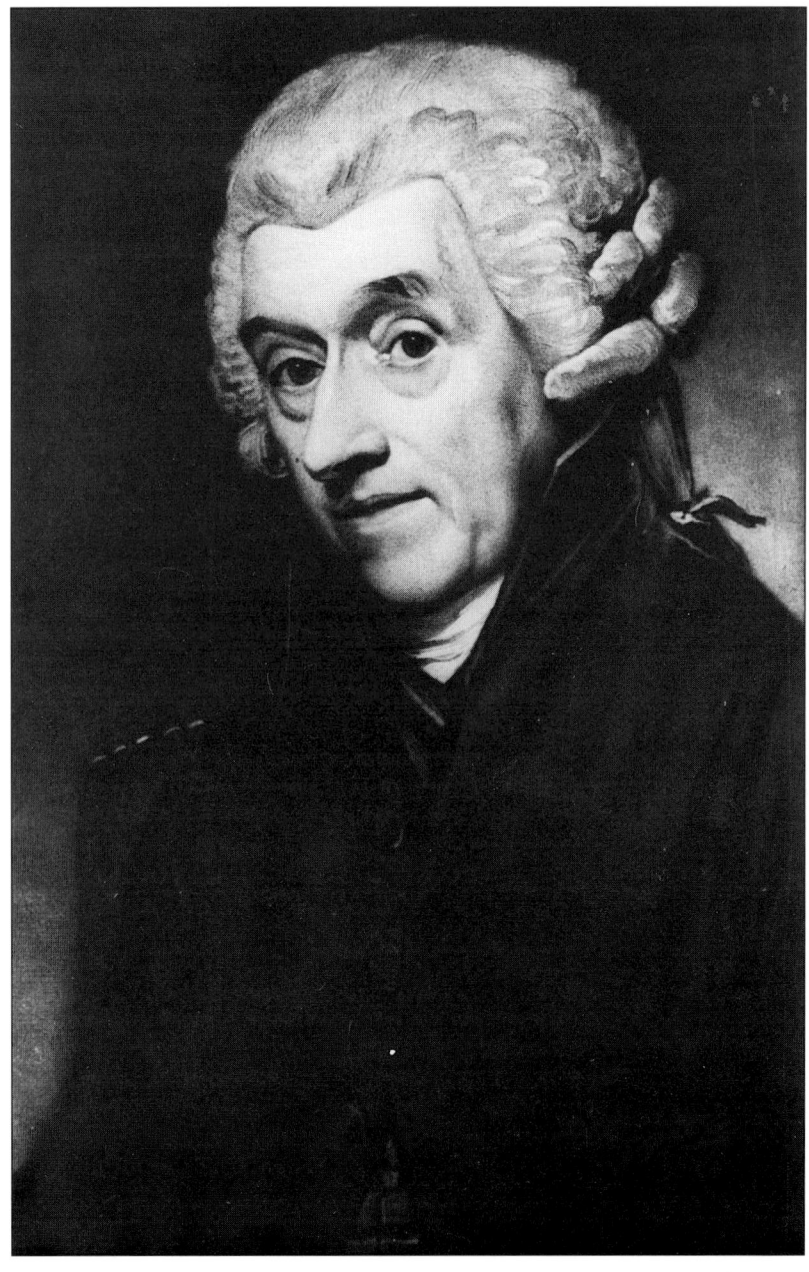

William Heberden. (Ernest Heberden, from William Heberden, *Royal Society of Medicine Services, 1989.)*

to mention a few of his achievements. In 1950 he was appointed Chairman of a governmental committee to report on the rheumatic diseases in which he had not previously shown great interest. Walking across from the College to the Athenaeum, I told him that if rheumatology did not now become better recognised he would have to take the blame. It was the only time I saw Henry truly shaken. It was the next year that he accepted the Presidency of the Heberden Society and in 1961 gave the Oration on William Heberden.

Matthew Ray, the first Chairman, came from Harrogate, where he was schooled in hydrotherapy. He served as Lt Col in World War I and with Fortescue Fox was an original member of the Peto Place Clinic.

Frank Howitt, the first President, was always involved in physical medicine. He received his CVO for the treatment of George V with actinotherapy and he was brought into the services in 1940 as Brigadier to form a team of physical medicine specialists for the army. He chose six physician/rheumatologists; Hugh Burt, son of the Bath rheumatologist, Ian Duthie, later Professor, selected by Stanley Davidson to 'head' rheumatology in Scotland; myself, the only member of the team already in the army as a medical specialist; Patterson of Droitwich; Will Tegner of London; and Arthur Wesson who was both FRCP and FRCS. Howitt became a great friend to us all, though he and I disagreed after the war, when he wished rheumatology and rehabilitation to become synonymous.

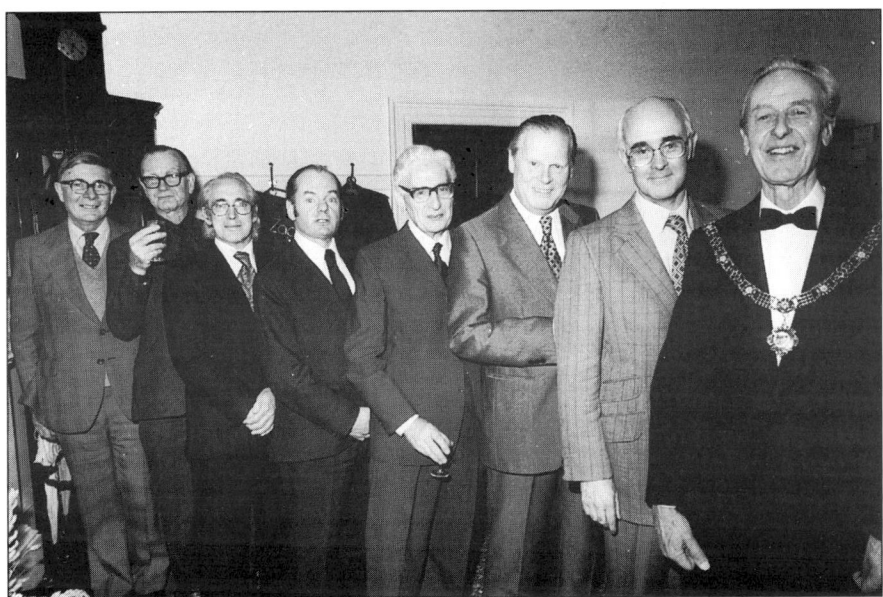

Seven Heberden Presidents, 1979.
Michael Andrews (Secretary), Eric Bywaters, John Ball, Allan Dixon, Leonard Glynn, 'Frank' Dudley Hart, Tom Scott, George Kersley.

While it would be quite inappropriate to give biographies in the text of all those who have helped to make the history of the Heberden Society, especially as these are available in full in Moll's excellent book, short biographies will be found in a separate chapter. However, a brief mention of a few not already discussed, helps to show how so many leaders of our profession have acted as Presidents and the names of the Orators demonstrate this society's international importance.

The early Presidents consisted of Frank Howitt, a leader in physical medicine, Matthew Ray originally from Harrogate, and then CB Heald who obtained a CBE in World War I and was interested in positive health as well as rheumatism. CB Buckley of Buxton, born 1874, was one of the first spa medical men of the 1930s to adapt this practice to modern rheumatology and was Editor of both the Royal College of Physicians' *Reports on Rheumatic Diseases* and the early *Annals of the Rheumatic Diseases*. SL Higgs, orthopaedist at St Bartholomew's Hospital, was the only surgeon to become President. Then came Will Copeman, Lord Cohen and Lord Horder whose contributions to rheumatology have already been described. Sir Ronald Tunbridge (born 1906) was Professor of Medicine at

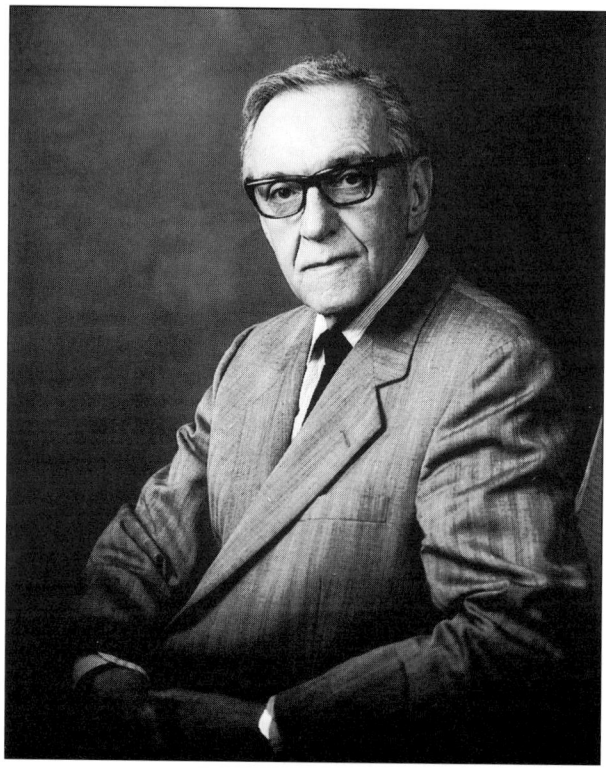

Morris Ziff. (Eric Bywaters)

Leeds; he served during the siege of Malta and was especially interested in the connective tissue diseases and cancer. Ernest Fletcher of the Royal Free and Arthur Stanley Institute was the first Heberden Orator. JH Kellgren became the first Professor of Rheumatology at Manchester after distinguishing himself in research at University College Hospital, 'Frank' Dudley Hart was Medical Consultant to the Westminster, as well as being in charge of rheumatology there. He was largely interested in therapy and his writings are still of great practical interest. Then came George Kersley of Bath and Eric Bywaters, the second physician to hold a Chair in Rheumatology, this time at the Postgraduate Medical School at Hammersmith Hospital. He was the 'Chief' Physician at Taplow and was one of rheumatology's most fertile early research brains.

Among the early Orators of international fame were Philip Hench, Hans Selye and Edward Kendall of cortisone and stress fame. Robert Stecher of Cleveland, Ohio, gave the oration in 1954 on Heberden Nodes and Genetics. Walter Bauer of Boston, a President of the American Medical Association was a great clinician, but persistently refused to accept that spondylitis was not just rheumatoid arthritis

Physical Medicine Section, Royal Society of Medicine, Dinner, 1941.

of the spine. Brochner-Mortensen of Copenhagen had a special interest in gout on which he gave his Oration. Charles Ragan of Columbia University and the Presbyterian Hospital New York gave his Oration on Hypersensitivity in the Pathogenesis of Rheumatoid Arthritis. Albert Neuberger from Warzburg, Germany, became Principal of the Wright Fleming Institute of Microbiology, London and did important work on connective tissue. Joe Bunim, born in 1906 in Russia, was later distinguished for his development of the National Institute of Arthritis and Rheumatic Disease at Bethesda. He gave his Oration on Sjogrens Syndrome. Jacques Forestier with his father Henri was a co-founder of La Ligue Contre le Rhumatism. They developed the gold treatment of rheumatoid arthritis, partly because of its clinical similarity to tuberculosis. In his youth Jacques was a great athlete of Olympic standard and throughout his life he maintained that youthful zest. In his latter years he described ankylosing vertebral hyperostosis sometimes known as 'Forestier's disease'. He worked partly in Paris, but mainly at his home town of Aix-les-Bains. Morris Ziff, latterly of Dallas, Texas, had a main interest in connective tissue diseases on which he gave his Oration in 1964. Since then there have been some twenty other distinguished Orators, whose names and dates are listed in the Appendix.

The Heberden Society remained the clinical 'heart' of rheumatology until 1984, when after much discussion it was amalgamated with the British Society for Rheumatism and Rehabilitation to become the British Society for Rheumatology (BSR). The name Heberden has however been retained for the Orators and Roundsmen.

The Royal Society of Medicine (RSM)
The RSM received its Royal Charter in 1834, took under its wing the British Balneological and Climatological Society in 1907 and this in its turn became the Physical Medicine Section of the RSM in 1931. By 1941, when I became President (GDK), more than half its interest was in rheumatology and in 1974 it followed the national trend and altered its name to the Section of Rheumatology and Rehabilitation. John Glyn became President 39 years later in 1970.

The Charterhouse Clinic
The Charterhouse Clinic was founded by a Dr Warren Crow as a rheumatology clinic, part of which was subsidised by public contributions. It was mainly known for its treatment with autogenous vaccines, based on the prevalent theory that all rheumatic conditions were due to infection. Organisms were obtained from the patient's teeth, gums, throat or bowel and were then made into a vaccine for administration. Though patronised by people in high places it was frowned on by the more orthodox members of the medical profession.

Our Hospitals in the 1930s
Apart from in London at Peto Place and later at St Stephen's and St John and Elizabeth in 1937 and the West London Hospital in 1938, most rheumatology was practised at the spas by the spa physicians. Buckley of Buxton stood out as one of the most eminent. Barnes Burt and Leslie Hill left Buxton for Bath where they played a very active role, Edgecombe and Yeomans, whose son later came to Bath as an orthopaedic surgeon, were working at Harrogate and Patterson at Droitwich. It was Bath however that led the way, when in 1936 the Royal Mineral Water Hospital changed its name to Royal National Hospital for Rheumatic Diseases to signify its dedication to treatment of arthritis.

References
1. Wells WC. Rheumatism and the Heart. *Trans Soc Improv Med Chir* 1812; **3**: 373.
2. Bouillaud JB. *Traite Clinique des Maladies du Cœur*. Paris: Baillière, 1835.
3. Aschoff L. Fur Myocarditisfrage. *Vehr Dtsch Ges Path*, 1904; **8**: 46.
4. Lancefield RC. Haemolytic Streptococci. *Harvey Lectures*, 1941; **36**: 251.
5. Garrod AB. Pathological conditions in blood and urine in gout. *Trans Med Chir Soc London*, 1848; **31**: 83.
6. Jennings GH. Use of salicylates as uricosurics in gout. *Rep Chr Rheum Dis* 1927; **3**: 106.
7. Talbott JH, Bishop C, Norcross BM, Lockie LM. Benemid in gout. *Trans Assoc Am Phys* 1951; **64**: 372.
8. Rundles RW, Wyngaarden JB, Hitchings GH. Effect of xanthine oxidase inhibition in gout. *Trans Assoc Am Phys* 1963; **76**: 126.
9. Seegmiller JE, Rosenbloom FE, Kelley WR. Enzymatic defect with excessive purine synthesis. *Science* 1967; **155**: 1682.
10. McCarty DJ, Hollander SL. Urate crystals in gouty synovial fluid. *Ann Intern Med* 1961; **54**: 452.
11. Sitaj S. Proc VI Congress Europ Rheum 1967: 547.
12. Dieppe PA, Huskisson EC. Apatitic deposition. *Lancet* 1976; **i**: 266.
13. Hench PS, Kendall EC, Slocumb CH, Polley HF. Effect of hormones on rheumatoid arthritis. *Proc Staff Mayo Clinic* 1949; **24**: 181.
14. Selye H. *J Clin Endocr* 1946; **6**: 117.
15. Klemperer P, Pollack AD, Bach G. Pathology of lupus erythematosus. *Arch Path*; **32**: 569.
16. Waaler E. Agglutination of sheep cell corpuscles. *Congress for Microbiology*. New York, Baltimore: Waverley Press 1940: 777.
17. Rose HM, Ragan C, Pearse E. Agglutination of sheep erythrocytes by sera of rheumatoid arthritis. *Proc Soc Exp Biol Med* 1948; **68**: 1.
18. Hargraves MM, Richmond H, Morton R. The tart cell and LE cell. *Proc Staff Mayo Clinic* 1948; **22**: 25.
19. Lilly F, Boyse EA, Old LJ. Genetic basis of leukaemogenesis. *Lancet* 1964; **ii**: 207.
20. Smith-Peterson MN. Arthroplasty of the hip. *J Bone Joint Surg* 1939; **21**: 269.

21 Judet J, Judet R. *Resection Reconstruction of Hip*. Edinburgh: London: E & S Livingstone, 1954.
22 Moore AT. Metal hip joint. *South Med J* 1952; **45**: 1015.
23 Charnley J. Anchorage of the femoral head prosthesis to the shaft of the femur. *J Bone Joint Surg* 1960; **42B**: 28.
24 Hendriksson RG *et al. Lancet* 1982; **ii**: 1395.

Chapter 3

The War Years

Throughout the country, as in previous wars, thoughts turned from rheumatology to rehabilitation of the wounded and injured. Frank Howitt, the late King's heliotherapist, was promoted Brigadier in charge of Physical Medicine in the army and he chose six physician/rheumatologists to head the team. Basil Kiernander and later Kit Wynn Parry were appointed to supervise physical medicine in the RAF and Frank Cooksey in the Civil Emergency Medical Services.

Physical medicine at that time was very different from what it is today. Working with the orthopaedists and army PT experts it was in charge of not only rehabilitation, but grading and advice on physical fitness, 'hardening off' and expert training of special services. In general it was responsible for advice on maintenance of 'cannon fodder'.

As an example of these diverse duties, when I (GDK) was changed from army medical specialist to physical medicine in Southern Command, I was told to reorganise the Army School of Physiotherapy at Netley and to open the first 'tough' school of Occupational Therapy at Taunton. Another of my duties was to vet, from the medical aspect, the Battle Schools, so that not too many men were broken in the training process. Again one had to examine the training of the

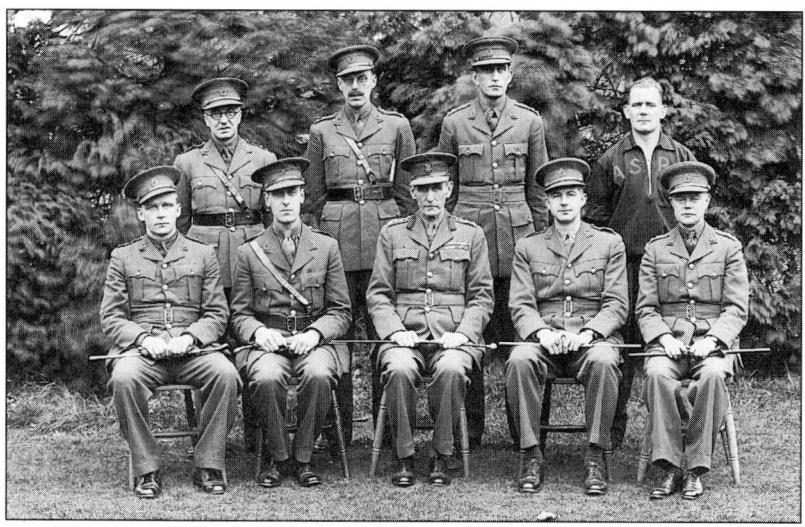

The British Army Physical Medicine Team, 1942.

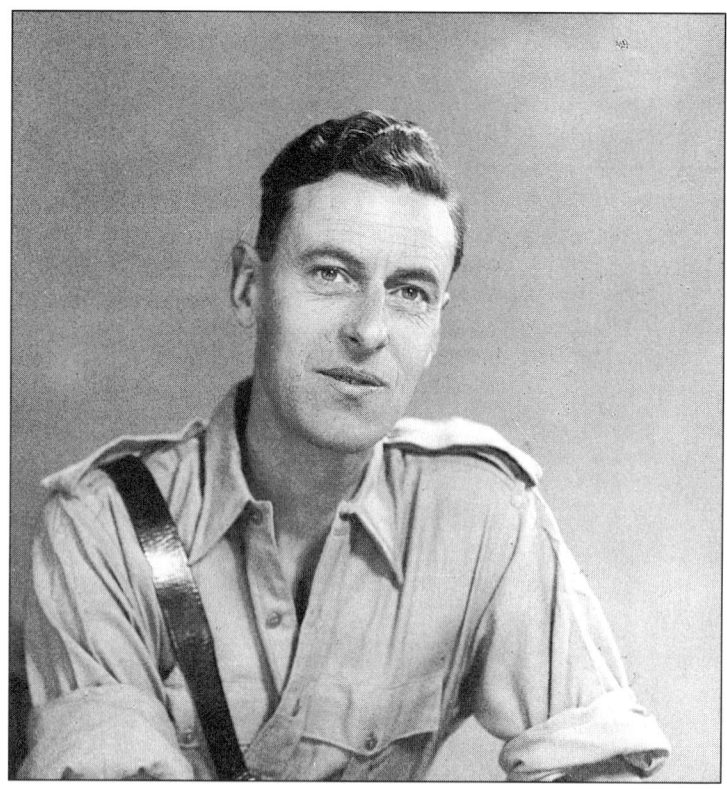

Col George Kersley, 1942, Adviser in Physical Medicine to Middle East.

paratroops to try to reduce the casualty rate of their drops and also to discuss the management of air sickness in towed aircraft. The work was very different from what I had imagined.

As the only physical medicine specialist selected for the team who was already in the services, I had been given the chance of objecting to the transfer. In 1940, however, expecting the war to finish in another six months, I thought some extra experience in rehabilitation would be of value when I returned to my real specialisation in the treatment of arthritis.

In 1942 I was promoted to Adviser in Physical Medicine to the Middle East Forces, with again a change in duties. On arrival at HQ in Cairo, I was summoned to see General Tomlinson, the DGAMS, a great and wise man who had seen the medical services through most difficult times. He told me he hadn't asked for me and knew nothing of my duties, but said I had better 'swan off' over my territory of Egypt, Palestine and Syria, and later including Persia and Iraq, and to report back in six weeks. Normally a consultant's reports were circulated and returned months later with comments from affected departments. I was however summoned at once before the DG who told me it was the most surprising report he had

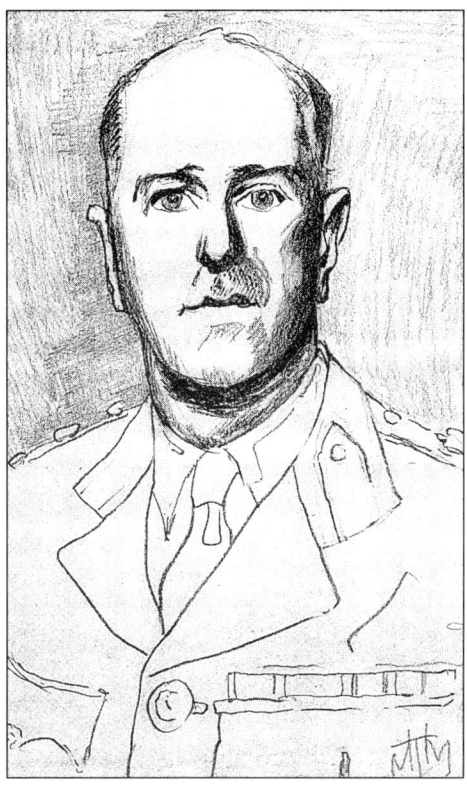

F D Howitt CVO, President of the Heberden Society. Leader of the Physical Medicine Team.

ever seen. He thought I was to give guidance on physiotherapy departments, but I had recommended the sacking of a Lieutenant Colonel, reorganising cooking arrangements and the building of a base cinema for a major Convalescent Depot. I replied that I believed my major priority was to turn five Convalescent Depots from 'concentration camps' into rehabilitation centres and save five thousand potential fighters from being invalided home by the psychiatrist. The Depots had been staffed by the discards of the combatant forces with a smattering of medical support and were seldom if ever visited by GHQ staff. By the time I returned home, two years later, all my suggestions had been agreed. They were not, however, popular with some of the 'medics', though supported enthusiastically by the A & G branches, who were in the main interested in 'cannon fodder' and the morale of those capable of returning to the lines. Of course I visited the physiotherapy departments of all military hospitals and helped to support the morale of the staff by, when possible, advising their transfers to the locality of their boyfriends! I was also in close touch with the BRCS in connection with their occupational therapy role.

After my return home, rather a bag of bones, I was given the job of sorting the unfit troops that had been sent to Northern Ireland into those to be discharged or who could be rehabilitated. While at Lisburne HQ, Belfast, rations were better than in England and in addition the RC padre used to tell me where to pick up butter, eggs and so on at farmhouses on my tour of so-called rehabilitation depots. On weekend leave I crossed the border to Eire, out of uniform of course, and here every luxury was available and everyone very friendly. Having been asked to bring back alcohol for the mess, I loaded my large suitcase with many bottles of gin, sherry and whiskey, covered the bottles with pyjamas and dressing gown and put one sherry bottle with cork drawn on top. To my surprise on the return journey the train was stopped for customs. My case was the first opened and I was told that they could not pass the sherry as a 'broken bottle'. I immediately suggested we passed it around the carriage. This provoked much laughter and I was told to close the case with no prying under my clothes. Everyone else in the carriage had their baggage turned out completely. I was very popular in the mess that night. My three months in Northern Ireland was almost like being out of the War.

The Irish Guiness consumed while playing liar dice with the Irish Director of Medical Services of an evening, sent me back to London District again fighting fit. The war was nearly over and, put up in the Guard's Mess at Knightsbridge and with perks like medical supervision of boxing by the services at the Albert Hall, life was quite pleasant.

One other assignment is worthy of mention, when I was loaned to the civil side for a couple of weeks to report on a new type of rehabilitation and resettlement unit at Sunningdale. I was afterwards called to Transport House, and I told them it was an excellent project, but that they should change the Director, who was only interested in wine and women. There was some consternation as I was told there was no post to which he could be promoted!

This description of my experience of physical medicine during the war gives some idea of the wide field of 'rehabilitation' at that time and which was so different from that in civil life.

The British Association of Physical Medicine (BAPM)

Shortly before I was posted overseas, in 1942, Lord Horder gave a lunch party at Claridges to which he invited the leaders in Physical Medicine from the Services, the EMS and the doyens of Harley Street, who had constantly been bickering and told them there was a war on and that they must get together and forget their personal rivalries.

Among those present were Sir Robert Stanton Woods, Sir Morton Smart, JB Mennell, Sir Frank Fox, Frank Cooksey, Francis Bach,

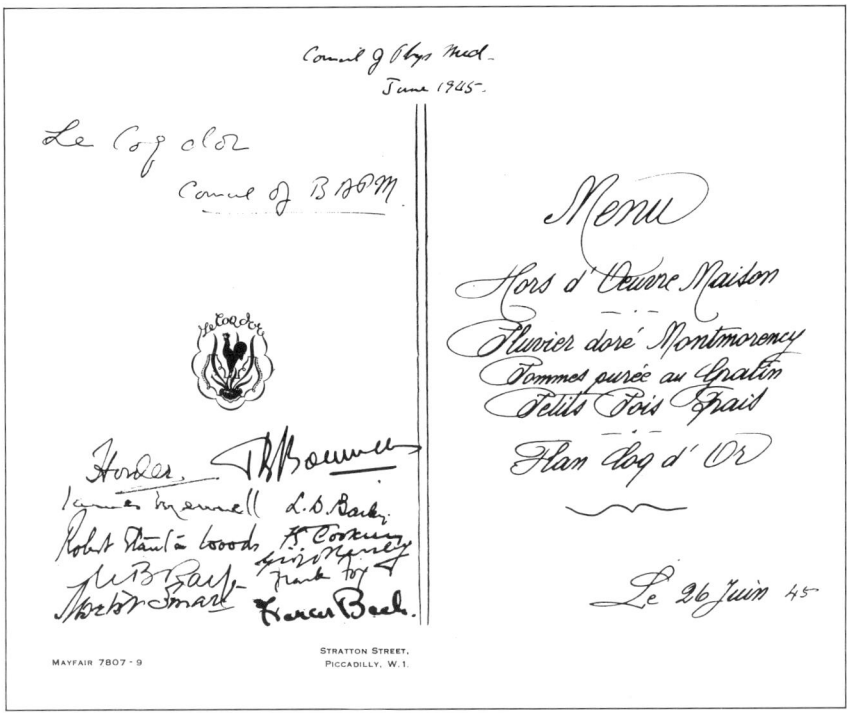

Signed menu of an early meeting of the British Association of Physical Medicine.

Matthew Ray, Phillipe Bauwens, LB Bailey, Brigadier Frank Howitt and some of his army team and Basil Kiernander and myself. JB Mennell was the father of medical manipulation, Phillipe Bauwens of medical electrotherapy and Frank Cooksey of the EMS Physical Medicine Services.

Seven months later, at a meeting at the Medical Society of London, the British Association of Physical Medicine, BAPM, was formed with Horder as the first President, Sir Morton Smart as Chairman and Phillipe Bauwens as Secretary.

After the War, in 1945, Frank Howitt became Chairman of the Association and its Headquarters then moved to the Royal College of Surgeons. In 1948 the College of Physicians instituted the Diploma of Physical Medicine and at the same time the NHS officially recognised the specialty. In 1952 it sponsored the first Congress of the International Federation of Physical Medicine at King's College in London.

The International Federation of Physical Medicine was first suggested at the International Congress on Medical Electronics held in Brussels in 1948 and a Committee was set up under the Chairmanship of Frank Krusen of Rochester, USA, with Clemmesen of Copenhagen as Vice Chairman. They asked the British Association of Physical Medicine (BAPM) to organise the first

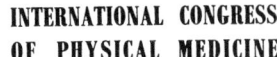

INTERNATIONAL CONGRESS OF PHYSICAL MEDICINE	OFFICIAL OPENING OF THE CONGRESS *by* Marshal of The Royal Air Force THE LORD TEDDER, G.C.B.
	Lighting of the Ceremonial Lamp
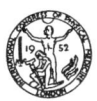	*Installation of the President of the Congress by the President of the Federation.*
	Speeches of Welcome: On behalf of H.M. Government The Rt. Hon. IAIN N. MACLEOD, M.P., Minister of Health On behalf of The International Federation of Physical Medicine Dr. FRANK H. KRUSEN (U.S.A.)
OPENING CEREMONY	Replies: Dr. S. CLEMMESEN (Denmark) Vice-Chairman, Interim Committee The International Federation of Physical Medicine Professor K. M. WALTHARD (Switzerland)
GREAT HALL, KING'S COLLEGE, STRAND, LONDON Monday, July 14th, 1952, 11 a.m.	Speech by The Rt. Hon. LORD HORDER, G.C.V.O. President, International Congress of Physical Medicine Vote of Thanks to LORD TEDDER by Dr. F. D. HOWITT, C.V.O.

First International Congress of Physical Medicine, 1952.

Congress in London in 1952 with Horder as President, Baruch and Krusen (USA), Bourgnignon (France), Clemmesen (Denmark), and Bauwens, Cooksey and Howitt (UK).

The Congress was opened by Lord Tedder with Lord Horder as President. The speakers were Iain Macleod, Minister of Health, Frank Krusen for the International Federation of Physical Medicine, Dr L Clemmesen (Denmark) and Professor Walthard (Switzerland). The Congress was followed by a visit to Oxford and the Spinal Injuries Centre at Stoke Mandeville established in 1944 and the Dorset House Occupational Therapy Centre, the first of its kind in the UK. Then there was a visit to Cambridge and the Papworth Village Settlement, founded for the resettlement of tuberculosis sufferers in 1916 and to Garston Manor opened in 1951 for 50 patients for three weeks' to three months' rehabilitation.

The official journal was at first the *Journal of Physical Medicine and Industrial Hygiene*, then the *Annals of Physical Medicine* and now the *Journal of Rheumatology and Rehabilitation*.

A detailed history of the BAPM is in the process of being written by Dr GO Storey and therefore its early history has only been summarised, though some of the problems it encountered over its overlap with rheumatology will be recorded in the next chapter.

In 1969 it changed its name by adding Rheumatology to its title and in 1973 it became the British Association of Rheumatology and Rehabilitation (BARR).

Chapter 4

The Post-War Period and the NHS

During the war the rheumatologists became rehabilitationists, but almost directly afterwards the internecine fighting between the two specialties broke out, made more confused by the onset of the NHS, which affected all the specialist hospital services. Let us therefore consider the effect generally of the NHS when it came into being in 1948.

The National Health Service
Bevan and the Labour Government seized the opportunity of post-war resettlement by bribing the many doctors who had been in the Forces for years, and in many cases for their whole career, by offering them a paid retraining period and assured future jobs under the new Beveridge plan. Every doctor was in agreement that a large extension of free medical care for all of the less well off and their dependants was necessary, but the sweeping change to include the wealthy in the service was unnecessarily revolutionary and caused some chaos. The very limited 'free' health service had been most unsatisfactory, with the need for dependants to belong to a Hospital Saving Association or Hospital Saturday Fund and for means testing by the hospital almoner. Many who required a consultation were too proud to go through this procedure and therefore requested a private opinion when they could not really afford it and this was traumatic both for consultant and patient. The sudden change from one extreme to the other however produced many problems. Many of the best GPs had country practices, where they looked after the poor of the village for very little or nothing, but also attended the nobility of the area for a reasonable fee. They now found that the Lord of the Manor, often living some distance from their home, expected the same service as before for the small NHS grant. They were expected to be available day or night and to wait while 'her Ladyship' completed her toilet before they were summoned to her room. In other, densely populated and poorer localities, there were streets packed with potential patients, who were accustomed to the doctor coming straight in and calling up the stairs to ask whether 'grannie's cough was less troublesome' and then off to the next house. These GPs became wealthy overnight.

Apart from this unfair effect on GPs' finances, the NHS drove a rift between its GPs and consultants. Before the NHS came into effect nearly all consultants did some general practice, while many GPs worked for higher examinations and then took up some sessions in their local hospital in a consultant capacity, as assistant physicians or surgeons. It is a pity that this grade disappeared, as it was in many ways the same status as that of our senior registrar today, but with security of tenure and the almost certain prospect of promotion to senior consultant in their hospital in due course.

Against this background we must consider the effect of the NHS on the fields of rheumatology and rehabilitation. In short it confused and blurred the distinction between the two specialties and jeopardised the future of the few hospitals specialising in the treatment of rheumatic disease.

When the NHS came into being, the rheumatologist was of course for the first time paid for his hospital work. He had, however, no registrar cover and was seldom reimbursed for his committee work or travel expenses for meetings abroad. The ARC tried to concentrate most of the committee meetings into one day per quarter—starting early and finishing late. League meetings and most other medical meetings meant cancelling clinics. With few rheumatologists we were very stretched. Apart from my clinical research commitments in Bath, I (GDK) had to cover Bristol with weekly clinics at the Bristol Royal and Southmead Hospitals and occasional visits to the rest of the South West and Oxford Regions.

There was little time for private work, but if one saw only a few private patients one's salary (and pension) was cut to nine elevenths. The pressure was such that I, perhaps foolishly, never took more than a half my entitlement of paid leave. It was all, however, a great challenge which one enjoyed. I was lucky in having three excellent but very different research assistants, paid for by grants. They attended my rounds and we met each week for a session on journals and literature and another for discussion of research projects. It was such a happy team that I had, after three years, to push them out to consultant posts elsewhere, one in the UK, one in Canada and one in the USA, as there were no internal prospects for them.

In view of the present NHS problems and hospitals possibly 'opting out', it is of interest to review the government of hospitals over the last seventy years, taking the Royal National Hospital for Rheumatic Diseases at Bath as an example.

Pre-war, all decisions were taken by the Committee of the Governors and on this sat the honorary staff consultants. As they were giving their services completely free and were the only members with medical knowledge, their recommendations were almost always agreed, provided the money to implement them could be found, mainly from private donations.

When the NHS initially took over all hospitals with their assets and debts, in most cases the latter, there was little interference from the local Health Authority except on very major matters of expenditure. In those days, as Chairman of the Medical Board, I met the Secretary and Matron once or twice a week over a cup of coffee and all decisions were easily agreed and ratified almost automatically by the Medical Board. Gradually however District Health Authorities began to interfere more and more, leaving little rope for local decision making. Reference of everything to District caused delays and often increased rather than reduced expenditure thus causing much frustration.

The 'opt out' of some hospitals to become independent trusts, still within the NHS, is part of the second revision of medical organisation by Government, against the advice of the BMA, who now claim that the NHS, which they opposed, is a sanctified success.

Once again many may feel that the reorganisation is precipitous, but it has been forced on the Government by the bottomless pit of financing the NHS, with the increased number of aging population, with fantastically expensive new treatments keeping the unfit alive longer, together with the demand of the public for more luxury in treatment facilities.

Utilising money to the greatest advantage and encouraging private participation, though unpopular, has become essential. At the same time it is necessary to insist on clinical and financial audit. In another decade a new NHS, perhaps after some bumps and minor modifications, will become the sacred cow the BMA now considers the present NHS to be.

The present suggestion of opting out will bring back more of the past independence and pride, though the District Authority and Region will still be responsible for seeing that patients have proper treatment and that the hospital is properly administered with a good accounting system. Funding will still be from the NHS, but the hospital will have more licence on how to use the money, provided it keeps within its budget.

The Royal National Hospital at Bath wishes to move out with its research centre to a site close to the large General (RUH) Hospital in order to be near the Wolfson Research Centre and the orthopaedic and paediatric departments, as well as to ease traffic problems and free the valuable site in the centre of the city. Opting out would guarantee that this specialist hospital was not absorbed into the RUH as has already been the case with the Orthopaedic Hospital and was suggested twenty years previously for the Royal National Hospital. Becoming just part of a general hospital complex would ruin its fantastic morale and do much to destroy its international status. It would certainly lose its Royal Coat of Arms only recently granted to it by the Queen.

The case for 'opting out' by the Royal National Hospital is perhaps rather exceptional, but many other hospitals are looking seriously at the value of having more independence, provided they can cope with the required administrative and audit reorganisation.

The internecine war—two views

1940-1950 (GDK)

Immediately after demobilisation, most of those who were originally physician/rheumatologists reverted to their previous interest. I resigned from the British Association of Physical Medicine, though a founder member. I did, however, rejoin two years later when I found that their members were producing useful research papers in my subject. Will Copeman, Eric Bywaters and others of the Hammersmith team were however most anxious not to become linked with the new physical medicine group, many of whom had not at that time the highest qualifications. At last the rheumatologist was becoming respectable and even more so after Phil Hench, the American Rheumatologist, obtained a Nobel Prize for the discovery of cortisone.

On the other hand my war-time chief Frank Howitt and Frank Cooksey of Kings College Hospital, who had built up the EMS rehabilitation service, were fighting hard to make the two specialties interchangeable, largely because it would gain for them hospital beds and a better chance in private practice. They were both personal friends of mine, but we were constantly having arguments on the matter.

One incident shows up the confusion and its augmentation by the NHS. As there were no registrars in rheumatology, Lord Horder led

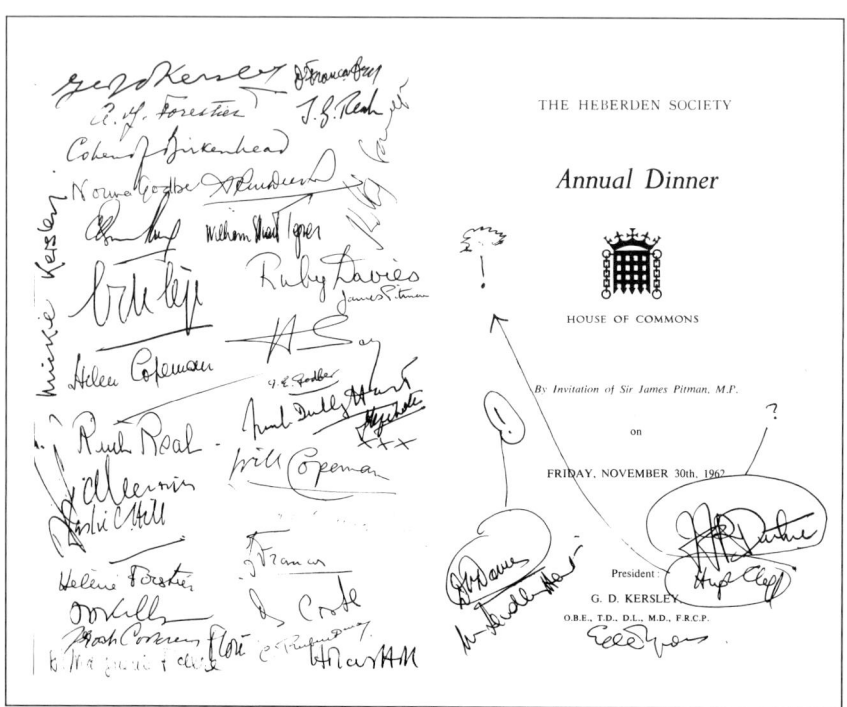

Heberden Society Dinner, 1962.

a delegation consisting of Will Copeman, Eric Bywaters and myself to the Ministry. We had a long session with Iain MacLeod, who eventually turned to his satellites saying we had a good case and asking why we had no registrars. They replied that we did have them, but they were called registrars in physical medicine!

Though firmly a 'rheumatologist', I was less of a hard liner than some. When President of the Heberden Society in 1962, I caused some consternation by pointing out in my speech at our Dinner in the House of Commons, that most of our members were also members of the BAPM and that half of the latter were in the Heberden Society. Was it not time we ceased to fight each other? Will Copeman and Eric Bywaters were not very pleased with my remarks.

Gradually the rift has narrowed, helped, as stated earlier, by the wisdom of the Royal College of Physicians who poured oil on the troubled waters.

The degree of specialisation was again a problem, as illustrated by my own case. I had always intended to remain a physician with a special interest in rheumatology, but when the NHS came into being I was given the difficult choice of remaining as I was or giving up my general medicine in order to start up the first Regionally funded Research Unit and act as Regional Adviser in Rheumatology, which at first covered the South West and Oxford areas. I opted for the latter course, but with much heart searching and at times regret, as I really loved my general medicine work.

At the same time there was a move to abolish specialist hospitals and incorporate them as small units in megolithic complexes of some 2000 beds.

The post-war ethos with regard to hospitals was that they should be large and contain wards or small departments to cover all specialties. Cardiff with its 2000 beds is a good example of such a complex. Such magnitude does however tend to stifle individuality and reduce corporate morale.

This cult, that big is beautiful, badly affected the Royal National Hospital at Bath. The outbreak of World War II had come eight days before the Queen was to lay the foundation stone of a new Royal National Hospital for Rheumatic Diseases on a new site by the river. It was to be for 220 beds with an orthopaedic department, theatre and nurses' home and the foundations had already been laid. All was postponed and after the war, though one corner of the old hospital had been hit by a bomb, the new building on what is now the Technical College site was again postponed. Having had our rebuilding assets seized in 1948, in 1954 we were told there would be no new hospital, that our old hospital was to be pulled down and the site sold. We were offered only a couple of wards at the RUH. My reply, as Chairman of the Medical Board, almost burnt the paper on which it was written. We immediately organised a deputation, which included the Mayor of Bath, the Chairman of the Regional

Board and the Vice Chancellor of Bristol University, to see the Minister of Health, but with no effect. Then ensued a battle lasting five years, the Region saying that as over half our patients came from outside their territory, we were not their responsibility, while the Ministry stated that there was no such thing as a national specialist hospital and that the Region was wholly responsible. I then burned my boats and gave a national press conference at the Royal College of Surgeons, an unheard of step in those days. It produced a fantastic response from every national paper. A week later Lord Tweedsmuir, President of the British Rheumatism Association, invited me to speak at an all party dinner of MPs in the House of Lords to explain our case for survival. Next day I heard from Sir George Godber that we had won, but that if we wanted a new research floor we must raise £20,000, in those days a lot of money. We succeeded and in 1965 Princess Marina, our Patron and throughout our campaign a great support, reopened our rebuilt hospital.

1949-1990 (JHG)
To label 1949 as the *Annus mirabilis* of rheumatology might suggest hyperbole, but there cannot be any doubt that many highly significant developments, both scientific and political date from around that time.

First and foremost, came the announcement in September 1949 at the International Congress of Rheumatology held in New York, that certain corticosteroids were dramatically able to reverse many of the acute manifestations of rheumatoid inflammation. No matter what therapeutic disappointments and frustrations were to beset us later, the proof that rheumatoid inflammation was potentially reversible attracted interest from scientists and clinicians with a wide diversity of interests and skills and this enabled basic research into the rheumatic diseases to develop as never before.

Secondly, it was at about this time that the concept that several rheumatic diseases might have a common basis related to abnormalities in the connective tissues was being propagated by Klemperer and Baehr.

The understanding of immunological processes was also expanding rapidly, particularly the concept of auto-immune processes as an explanation of the perpetuation of rheumatic inflammation, long after the initial insult had passed.

In Canada, Hans Selye, was publishing his alluring theories based on impressive experiments, which related stress to disease in several animal models, including adjuvant arthritis in rats. According to his theory, this reaction was mediated via the pituitary-hypothalamic adrenal axis, thereby possibly linking with the therapeutic benefits of the glucocorticoids and corticotrophin, which had been recently described.

This work on the connective tissue diseases led to the formation of two schools of thought, known colloquially as the 'lumpers' and the 'splitters', those who believed either that there was a condition of 'collagen disease' with various manifestations or that each syndrome was a separate disease. Some of the complex metabolic disorders of purine metabolism associated with the arthritis of gout were becoming clearer. Largely as the result of observations made on the armed forces during the war, many new and important advances occurred in the understanding and management of ankylosing spondylitis. This led to a radically altered programme of management by active exercises and other forms of rehabilitation

In summary, these were exciting times for anyone who decided to specialise in a subject that hitherto had been uniformly thought of as a 'Cinderella' specialty.

It was into this plethora of exciting developments that I entered the field, on September 1st 1949. The mode and reason for my decision to specialise in rheumatology were, to say the least of it, providential. Suffice it to record that I was employed as a research registrar on a unit designed to search for possible analogues to cortisone, and to be prepared to carry out the necessary clinical observations if and when cortisone itself became available in this country.

On this last point, there was still room for doubt, if only because of the immense production difficulties encountered by the chemists at Merk Sharpe and Dohme (which was the only pharmaceutical company attempting its production at that time). As an example, the technical complexity of adding an oxygen and a hydroxyl group at the eleventh and the seventeenth positions of the basic steroid nucleus, respectively, had not been solved, at least on a commercial basis. Secondly, the only known starting point of production—namely the bile of cattle—seemed likely to remain in permanently short supply. In a noble attempt to overcome this supply problem, Messrs MSD created what became virtually a monopoly market for cattle and sheep gall bladders throughout the USA much to the surprise and pleasure of the farmers, who were suddenly enabled to sell a previously useless viscus. This created a remarkable Black Market in the USA where patients, having learned of the new 'wonder drug', were willing to pay grotesquely inflated prices to obtain a supply, frequently for the treatment of inappropriate diseases.

In those days they were using inflated dosages, without appreciating the potentially serious side-effects, and many became totally dependent on (and possibly addicted to) corticosteroids. This resulted in a great problem for their physician when an attempt was made to wean them. The weaning process was always long and painful; it was also frequently unsuccessful and the tragedies produced were compounded of sociological and psychological as well as pharmacological aspects.

In contrast, the British government's approach of strictly limiting imports to genuine research projects at least eliminated similar problems in the UK.

I worked on this research unit for two to three years; then obtained a fellowship in the academic study group on rheumatic diseases at the New York University medical school. These experiences, not unnaturally, stimulated my interest in the specialty of rheumatology and I returned from the USA, determined to continue my training as a rheumatologist.

It was at this point that I first encountered the career problems that were to beset my generation of rheumatologists for the next thirty-three years.

The problems arose partly as the result of the massive demobilisation of doctors from the armed forces, as well as those who had been conscripted at the end of the war for their mandatory two years' service. The former were guaranteed hospital training posts in the newly developing NHS. This was under an edict from Aneuran Bevan the Minister of Health. If necessary, supernumerary registrar posts were to be created to accommodate the inflated numbers.

At the end of their training, however, no extra consultant posts were made available to accommodate those who wished to continue their specialist careers in hospital work. This inevitably resulted in an awesome 'bottle-neck' on the final rung of the training ladder, ie established consultant posts.

In such circumstances, it is hardly surprising that new and developing specialties such as rheumatology tended to be relegated to the back of the queue. Indeed, in 1949 the career prospect for a fully trained rheumatologist was negligible, and, with the exception of a very few university appointments, this situation continued for about seven years.

Because of the requirements of the armed services during the war for efficient rehabilitation services, the specialty previously known as physical medicine had burgeoned into an expanded and highly regarded branch of the armed forces medical services. The doctors placed in charge of these units were either orthopaedic surgeons, or they were physicians whose civilian experience had been concerned with the treatment of musculo-skeletal disorders, mainly by physical methods. The significance of physical methods at that time was, of course, related to the virtual absence of any effective drug therapy except for aspirin.

After the war, it became the policy of the Ministry of Health, that, wherever possible, ancillary medical departments such as those of physiotherapy and occupational therapy should be under the administrative and clinical supervision of a doctor. Not unnaturally, it was to the rehabilitation specialists from the armed services that they turned for this supervision. A few new consultant posts in physical medicine were created with this objective in view.

The incumbents of these posts frequently felt they should take full clinical responsibility for the care of patients with rheumatic diseases and they could not understand why a further group of specialist rheumatologists was required.

By contrast, those who had opted for an exclusive training programme in rheumatology were offering a full-time commitment to rheumatology, which they felt was vital if the status of the subject was to improve and, above all, become acceptable to the rest of the profession and the medical schools. They also offered a parallel commitment to promote clinical and basic research into the pathophysiological mechanisms of this much neglected group of diseases. Finally, they accepted responsibility for the setting up and implementation of training programmes for future generations of rheumatologists. It was felt that only by these measures could British rheumatology compete with the increasingly sophisticated developments occurring at that time in the USA and indeed in Europe.

The third and fourth groups who claimed responsibility for the clinical care of rheumatological patients were the general physicians and the orthopaedic surgeons. Traditionally, general physicians had accepted most of the rheumatological patients referred to hospital for a consultation in their general medical clinics, and this seemed satisfactory, apart from the problems of long-term follow up and the co-ordination of the social and ancillary treatment services. Many general physician colleagues were bitterly opposed to the setting up of yet another medical specialty service. At the most, they argued, all that was needed was for one general physician in each district hospital to interest himself in this group of diseases in the course of his general medical duties.

Orthopaedic surgeons had a specialised interest in the prevention and treatment of established deformities. Most of them were too busy to accept full clinical responsibility and were satisfied by the collaboration of their physician colleagues, especially those who were willing to set up joint clinics to monitor patients of mutual interest.

What the rheumatologists could not accept, was the implication that they should take responsibility for the running of the physio/occupational and other ancillary therapeutic departments. This became a major bone of contention, not only with professional colleagues, but also with the Ministry. In some cases the proposed 'umbrella' responsibilities would extend to speech therapy and orthotic departments. Almost invariably they included responsibility for providing the electro-diagnostic services of the hospital.

Rheumatologists argued that the acceptance of these additional responsibilities would greatly dilute their capacity to nurture the scientific and clinical aspects of this 'Cinderella' specialty and would certainly mitigate against the professional acceptance of the subject as having similar status to the parallel specialties of, for example, neurology and cardiology, both of which were by this time fully accredited under the umbrella of general medicine. Furthermore, it cannot be denied that the psychological prejudices voiced by, admittedly prejudiced, academics against 'light shiners' and other perjorative terms, had to be expunged if there was to be any hope of the specialty of rheumatology being taken seriously.

The obverse argument arose from those who felt that the subject of rehabilitation was of itself an underdeveloped specialty which would benefit from the wisdom of full-time specialists, who would devote their talent to planning improvements in a service which, it was argued, was only marginally concerned with the rheumatic diseases (and even then only the chronic and crippling cases).

Therefore, it was argued that a specialist in charge of rehabilitation might equally appropriately be a neurologist, an orthopaedic surgeon, a cardiologist or even a chest physician, all of which specialties were utilising to an increasing extent the services of rehabilitation departments for their patients. As an example of the problem, one only needed to cite the case of paraplegia, where modern management required a high degree of sophistication and training, which the average rheumatologist would feel completely incompetent to provide. The same argument would apply to the esoteric developments in the field of electro-diagnosis, which had long since outstripped the simple intensity/duration curves with which most of us were familiar. Such developments rendered the concept of a 'Pooh-Bah' director of rehabilitation services completely outmoded.

It will therefore be appreciated that the future of the rheumatological services under the NHS stood at great risk of becoming hopelessly fragmented. Characteristically, where the NHS was concerned, there was a strong *economic* argument in favour of combining the appointments of specialists in rheumatology with the responsibility of the rehabilitation services. Because the Ministry of Health was effectively a monopoly employer of the hospital services throughout the UK, the future of the specialty rested very much in their hands. The only alternative potential sponsors were the few university medical schools who could be persuaded to fund a research programme and the ERC, whose limited budget confined its sponsorship to one or two strategically situated professorships. It was hoped that these would act as 'flagships' for future developments.

Private and pharmaceutically funded research projects were exceedingly rare (although my own fellowship on the cortisone research unit was in fact funded by the manufacturers of Cherry Blossom boot polish to their eternal credit!).

It was in this manner that the stage was set for rivalry, and indeed feuding, between two groups whose clinical objectives—namely the management and welfare of sufferers from rheumatic diseases—should have coincided. Both groups claimed that they were approaching rheumatological problems from a clinical standpoint, and both demanded an acceptable higher degree before recognising consultant status. In the case of the physical medicine group, however, several colleagues had achieved consultant status before these mandatory training standards were introduced. Some of these did not measure up to the criteria of clinical experience, which both groups felt were essential. This minority group constituted a bone of contention which further increased the rivalry. It was a problem which could only be solved by the passage of time.

One striking aspect of the feuding years was the capriciousness of the situation. One's loyalties were largely related to where one was trained. Those with research interests and skills naturally gravitated towards the academic units of rheumatology. Those of us whose primary career interests were in the field of clinical research or clinical practice were compelled to take a more eclectic approach relating to the prospects of achieving consultant status within the NHS in the foreseeable future.

Personal friendships and respect between colleagues in the rival groups were commonplace, and the increasingly common membership of both professional societies (The Heberden Society and the British Association of Physical Medicine) brought us together at clinical and academic meetings. However, in political terms, any suggestion of a fusion into a single group, representing both our interests, was sedulously resisted by both sides, and it is difficult to escape the conclusion that most of the resistance came from entrenched prejudices by the older hierarchies of both groups. Meanwhile, career aspirants on both sides felt seriously frustrated and, unhappily, many were forced to give up their training, or to emigrate.

Apart from the sources of friction already noted, it is difficult after this length of time to pinpoint all the other seemingly insoluble problems. One of them was certainly to do with the name of the specialty. To the rheumatologists, the title of 'physical medicine', was both opprobious and irrelevant to their primary objectives. The rival group however seemed curiously wedded to it, and apart from a willingness to add the word 'rehabilitation' to their title were quite unwilling to consider abandoning it.

Another divisive point was the examination called the Diploma of Physical Medicine, which, although not mandatory, was considered as being desirable for those applying for consultantships. This examination demanded amongst other subjects a seemingly useless study of physics which, to the rheumatologists, was symptomatic of physical medicine's concern with machines. It also involved a moderately intensive study of musculo-skeletal anatomy which I have found useful in subsequent practice. The examination was eventually abandoned in favour of one called Diploma of Medical

Rehabilitation, thereby reflecting a change in emphasis and interest.

In retrospect, the quarrels between the two groups may sound trivial and futile, indeed many of them were. However, for those who were trained during that era, they were immensely real and the source of much anxiety. They were not finally solved until 1984, ie a full thirty-five years after the establishment of the NHS. In that year, the Heberden Society was wound up and merged with the British Association of Rheumatology and Rehabilitation (as the BAPM had been renamed in 1970) the combined society being called the British Society for Rheumatology. The events leading to this merger are dealt with elsewhere.

It is interesting to relate these events to the parallel developments of the two professional societies which sought to represent the seemingly disparate interests of the rheumatologists and those whose primary concern was in physical medicine. Although these societies inevitably had a large common membership, they grew up entirely independently and with strikingly divergent rules and philosophies.

Essentially the interests of the Heberden Society were confined to clinical and basic sciences which might have a bearing on the rheumatic diseases. It was limited to one hundred full members, with a slightly larger associate membership. In order to be elected as a full member, it was mandatory to read a paper for approval before the Society. They elected an annual 'Orator' and an annual 'Heberden Roundsman', both of which were, and indeed still are, regarded as prestigious appointments. Virtually all of the members had higher degrees in medicine, such as an MRCP or an MD, others were those engaged in full-time basic research. Reciprocal contacts with foreign societies were encouraged and the obtaining of training fellowships with overseas units was strongly supported, and appropriate introductions facilitated.

The British Association of Physical Medicine was by contrast essentially a clinical society, with a versatile range of interests, primarily in musculoskeletal and neurological diseases. Within the field of rheumatology its interests, although widespread, tended to concentrate on the hinterland between orthopaedic surgery and what was called, by at least one group (Dr Cyriax's Group at St Thomas's Hospital), 'orthopaedic medicine'. This term not only included the vexed problems presented by backache care, but it also referred to the diagnosis and treatment of periarticular and soft tissue conditions. Such syndromes had previously tended to be neglected, if only because responsibility for their management had been fragmented between different departments.

This is not to imply that physical medicine specialists were incapable of, or disinterested in, looking after the more serious collagen/vascular diseases, but merely that their clinical 'catchment' tended to be overburdened with the commoner, but less serious, variety of rheumatic illnesses.

The concept of rehabilitation was nebulous in these early days including, as it did, not only 'physical' rehabilitation but also social and community responsibilities. Such aspects nowadays tend to be carried out by a community physician, but in those days they were accepted as an important part of the responsibility of physical medicine specialists.

Another eclectic responsibility accepted by the physical medicine group in the early days was that of electrodiagnosis. Indeed, there was at least one hospital unit (Dr Bauwen's group of St Thomas's Hospital) whose interests and expertise virtually excluded other activities.

Gradually, as the sophistication of electronic equipment increased, the responsibility for these investigations came to be shared between those physical medicine colleagues who retained a special interest, neurologists and neurosurgeons.

The situation described in the UK was becoming increasingly divergent from that in the USA and many European countries where there already was a complete dissociation between the specialties of rheumatology, physical medicine and rehabilitation; these discrepancies started to create increasing difficulty in any attempted association with our foreign counterparts, with corresponding difficulties experienced by those who wished to carry out part of their training overseas.

Chapter 5

Participants in Post-War Developments

Hospital developments

After World War II, departments dealing with rheumatology, rehabilitation and bone disease gradually became established, often with ARC support. The London Hospital requires special mention for its Bone and Joint Unit, where Harry Currey and Michael Mason were particularly involved. The latter's name has therefore been perpetuated by the Michael Mason Prize, since his sudden tragic death in 1976 during the ILAR Conference in San Francisco, where he was serving as BLAR President.

The Canadian Red Cross Hospital, Taplow

In 1947 the Canadian Red Cross established a unit for the Study of Juvenile Rheumatism at Taplow under the leadership of Eric Bywaters. He had previously been at the rheumatology unit at Hammersmith Postgraduate Hospital, to which my (GDK) old chief Sir Francis Fraser had moved from St Bartholomew's Hospital. Eric Bywaters, born in 1910, trained at the Middlesex Hospital, moved to Hammersmith in 1940 and became Professor of Rheumatology there in 1958. This was the second Chair to be established in the UK. It was only preceded in 1953 by a Chair in Manchester held by Jonas Kellgren. Eric was joined by Barbara Ansell and together they made Taplow world famous in the field of paediatric rheumatology.

The Kennedy Institute

In 1961, a foundation gift of £500,000 was made to the Charing Cross Hospital Group by the Mathilde and Terence Kennedy Charitable Trust for the purpose of creating the first 'purpose built' institute, designed specifically for combined laboratory and clinical research into the cause of the rheumatic diseases. It was housed adjacent to the West London Hospital, where there already existed a flourishing clinical rheumatology unit, under the direction of Drs Will Copeman and Oswald Savage. The building was completed and officially opened in October 1966. The provenance of the funds for this important development is of some interest. Mathilde Kennedy was the daughter of Michael Marks, the founder of the Marks and Spencer empire. She suffered from arthritis of her hip, and was a patient of Copeman's. However, it appears that her

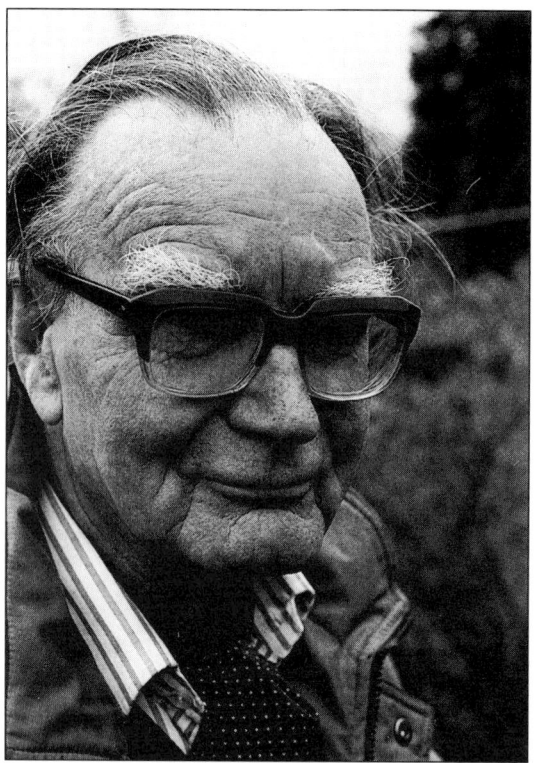

Professor Eric Bywaters. (Eric Bywaters).

particular interest in helping rheumatism research arose from her distress at witnessing the rapid and inexorable crippling of her GP, for whom she had a particular respect and affection, from polyarthritis.

The Spinal Injuries Centre, Stoke Mandeville
Ludwig Guttmann was originally a neurosurgeon in his native Germany, where he qualified at Freiburg in 1924. He came to the UK gaining a British qualification in 1939. He became associated at Oxford, with Sir Hugh Cairns, who, during World War II, ran the Army's Head Injury Unit. In due course Guttmann was asked to take charge of the rehabilitation of those whose injuries had resulted in paraplegia. Previous attempts to treat and rehabilitate such patients had proved frustratingly unrewarding and the victims usually succumbed quickly to irreversible infection and renal failure. Undeterred, Guttmann accepted his brief, and his intelligence and persistence wrought a virtual revolution in the

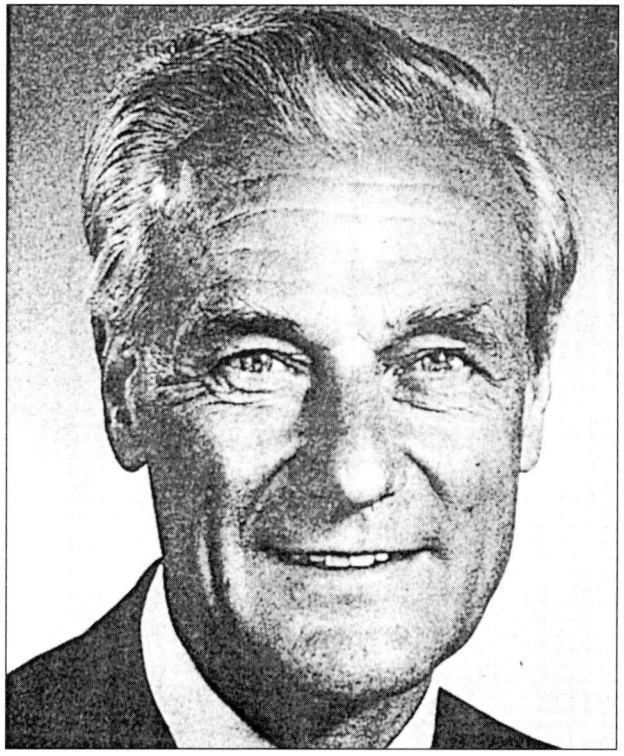

Professor Jonas Kellgren.

management of this condition. Even more remarkable, however, was the dramatic change in morale which he was able to induce in the Spinal Injuries Centre at Stoke Mandeville Hospital which he founded in 1944.

The introduction and development of the Paraplegic International 'Olympic Games' is of itself a sufficient testimony to his remarkable foresight and pioneering zeal. For his contribution to neurological rehabilitation and establishment of Stoke Mandeville as an international centre he received a knighthood.

The centre became associated with the Star and Garter Home, London and Chaselycot at Eastbourne, the Duchess of Gloucester Hospital at Isleworth, Lyme Green Hall at Macclesfield and Koytes Estate at Watford to all of which patients were transferred.

Patient involvement

In the post-war decade there were two other factors, apart from the effect of the NHS and the confusion over specialisation, that influenced rheumatology very greatly. Firstly the previously described discovery of cortisone and of the effects of stress by teams interested in rheumatology in America and Canada, which had a great influence on the attitude of the academics to the specialty. Secondly the upsurge of self help groups and the realisation of the importance of welfare services in treatment has made a great impact.

Although the Diabetic Association had been in existence for some years, the first self help group in the rheumatic field was the British Rheumatism Association, followed more recently by the formation of the Spondylitis Society and Systemic Lupus groups.

The British Rheumatism Association (Arthritis Care)
The British Rheumatism Association (BRA), later becoming the British Rheumatism and Arthritis Association (BRAA) and now Arthritis Care, was founded in 1947 by a solicitor, AC Bowen, who was a sufferer. Its objectives were to get together arthritics to help and support each other and to exert pressure to obtain better treatment services. Lord Nuffield was their first President, followed by the Hon Angus Ogilvie in 1963. Subsequent Presidents were Lord Tweedsmuir and now the Duke of Westminster. In 1972 the Duke of Edinburgh became Patron till 1977, when the Hon Angus Ogilvie took over this office. Francis Bach was a Founder Member and their Medical Adviser, and Mrs Neville Rolfe was their Secretary. As mentioned before, Francis Bach and Will Copeman were not firm friends and Mrs Neville Rolfe, a rheumatoid arthritic and a most enthusiastic and hard working lady, was not the most tactful and easy person to work with. Thus rivalry, not co-operation, existed between the BRA and the ARC.

When Horder and I (GDK) joined the BRA it was not with the approval of the ARC. We, however, felt that somehow the ARC and BRA should be working in parallel. The latter being a non-medical body dealing only with welfare, should not impinge on the work of the ARC on research and teaching. Gradually the ill feeling has decreased and there is now closer co-operation. At branch level, for instance at Bath, the two executive committees have each asked the other to nominate a representative.

For some years Dr Douglas Woolf and the late Dr Logie Bain did a great deal to help this more happy state of affairs, especially since the former became Chairman.

The Association, now with Regional Directors and local Branches, runs excellent homes and holiday centres, a correspondence service and a very good informative quarterly paper.

The Horder Homes
The Horder Homes were founded in 1964 at Crowborough in East Sussex to provide residential accommodation for the physically

handicapped. Lord Horder was their first President and, after his decease, was followed by Princess Margaret. Miss Cecilia Bochenek was the power behind the scene when the Horder Homes opened with 18 beds, and for many years afterwards. There are now 36 beds and Dr Douglas Woolf has taken over as part-time Medical Director and Consultant.

The back pain association and society

The study of back pain was neglected for many years, probably for the same reason that rheumatology was neglected twenty years before—because it was so widespread and difficult to define, and because treatment was largely in the hands of unqualified practitioners or cranks. So where to start?

In 1960 the Institute of Directors recognised the economic importance of back pain and sponsored the formation of the Back Pain Association. Lord Wall became chairman with Admiral Sir Caspar John and Mr Stanley Grundy as his henchmen. Dr Beric Wright became their Medical Adviser, Miss Sadler, Secretary and Sir Richard Powell was elected President.

In 1971 the Association sponsored a medical and scientific meeting at the Bath Institute of Medical Engineering, at which the Back Pain Society was formed with Dr Allan Dixon as its first chairman. Its objectives were the interchange of scientific information and research leaving the Association the role of propaganda and fund raising. The Association's journal *Talk Back* has proved a great success. It has also, with the help of Rotary, started Back Pain Groups throughout the country for sufferers and those interested in back pain, to promote mutual help and fund raising.

Similar to these groups are the branches of the National Ankylosing Spondylitis Society (NASS), originally developed for self-assistance of patients from the Royal National Hospital for Rheumatic Diseases at Bath. Likewise there is now a flourishing group of systemic lupus erythematosus sufferers.

The British Association of Manipulative Medicine

Manipulation has been used by non-medical bone setters, osteopaths and chiropractors for many years. In the early 1930s JB Mennell of St Thomas's Hospital taught the value of simple manipulation, especially for movements not under voluntary control, to his physiotherapists and doctors. It was not, however, until 1963 that members of the medical profession, many also qualified in osteopathy or chiropractic, came together to form the British Association of Manipulative Medicine. Their objectives were improvement of, and exchange of knowledge about manipulative and injection techniques used in locomotor medicine. Like the rheumatologists and physical medicine specialists before them, they had a tough job in becoming recognised as a reputable body. They even had to start by trying to learn a common language, as their terminology and theory was often divergent. Three of us who worked at major hospitals, but were not involved in manipulation, attended their early meetings to try and give encouragement and guidance. For full and proper use to be made generally of this important therapy, it was necessary to persuade the academics to include a modicum of it in the undergraduate curriculum. Their first President was Dr Barbor, followed by Dr Cyriax, then succeeded by Dr John Ebbetts, their earlier Secretary, and now by Dr John Davidson.

The National Osteoporosis Society
Osteoporosis is now closely associated with rheumatology especially in its relationship to degenerative joint disease and the iatrogenic effect of steroids. The National Osteoporosis Society for research and treatment of this condition was founded in 1986 under the chairmanship of Alan Dixon at Redstock.

The National Ankylosing Spondylitis Society (NASS)
This society, with its headquarters in London and under the directorship of Mr Rogers, arose out of a group of spondylitics who were regularly admitted for treatment at the Royal National Hospital for Rheumatic Diseases at Bath. It was founded in 1975 and has played a large part in the formation of the Ankylosing Spondylitis International Federation in 1988.

Other groups
Other groups are gradually coming into being, such as that of systemic lupus sufferers under the leadership of Graham Hughes.

Chapter 6

American Rheumatology and Physiatry

Developments in the United States of America

Rheumatology
In 1927, ten prominent physicians with an interest in rheumatology formed themselves into a group which they called The American Committee for the Control of Rheumatism, under the chairmanship of Dr Ralph Pemberton. This soon became affiliated with the International League against Rheumatism.

In 1932 the group organised its first scientific meeting in New Orleans, and a perusal of the subjects chosen for discussion makes fascinating and quaint reading, reflecting as they do current hypotheses and practises. Conversely it is salutary to appreciate that one or two of the subjects discussed on that first occasion remain topical in our own contemporary meetings—for example an attempt to classify degenerative arthritis.

Early in 1934 the original committee formed themselves into an association which they named The American Association for the Control of Rheumatism (the name also appears in contemporary papers as The American Association for the Study and Control of Rheumatic Diseases).

One of the early activities of this Association was to institute reviews of international literature, to be updated at frequent intervals. These *Rheumatism Reviews* as the series came to be known, continued to be published, until very recently, and represent an excellent 'bird's eye view' of the subject as it developed over the subsequent fifty years.

In 1937 the Association was re-named The American Rheumatism Association (ARA), a name which has lasted until now, and annual meetings were organised with a progressively wider and more sophisticated spectrum of subjects included for discussion.

From 1940 onwards meetings of the Association were disrupted by the impact of World War II, and indeed from 1942 until the end of the war there was a complete cessation of any formal meetings, largely because so many members and leaders of the ARA were in the armed forces. Five army hospitals were in fact designated to the care of military personnel who had rheumatic illnesses. It is an interesting reflection of disease coincidence at the time that three were for patients with rheumatic fever, and two for other forms of rheumatic diseases. On the professional staff of these army rheumatism centres were many prominent members of the ARA, who thus maintained some interest in the rheumatic diseases during the preoccupations of the war. Despite the war-time disruption, the ARA grew steadily in its membership, numbering 226 in 1940 and 260 in 1944. A few arthritic research centres were established, and medical colleges began to include arthritis in their teaching curriculum. Regional rheumatism societies were formed in some of the larger cities.

The first post-war 'reunion meeting' of the Association was held in June 1946 in New York City, and the first post-war President was Dr Paul Holbrook of Arizona, who was succeeded in 1946 by Dr Walter Bauer.

An education and research committee was set up in 1947 and fund raising started in earnest under the auspices of a powerful lay and professional organisation. Efforts were made to co-ordinate all fund raising into an international fund, named the American Rheumatism Foundation, which first met in New York in May 1948. Meanwhile the multiplicity of local fund-raising associations, which had sprung up independently, were encouraged to merge and co-operate with the national organisation, and with few exceptions they agreed to do so. It was agreed initially that eleven regional Chapters should continue to act under the aegis of the National Foundation. The first annual meeting was held in New York City in May 1949, shortly before the Seventh International Congress, at which—as already noted—the Mayo Clinic Group announced their startling observations on the anti-inflammatory potential of the corticosteroids.

During the 1940s and especially in the early post-war years, the US Public Health Service issued several reports describing the magnitude and importance of rheumatic diseases as a major health problem, and armed with the facts a campaign for Government support for research into arthritis and rheumatism gathered momentum.

Resulting from this pressure, a Bill was introduced to Congress in January 1949 designed to support research and training in the rheumatic diseases, and to aid the various States in the development of community programmes for the control of these diseases. The Bill called for the establishment of a National Arthritis and Rheumatism Institute in the Public Health Service, and for the appointment of a National Advisory Arthritis and Rheumatism Council to assist a Surgeon General in carrying out the purposes of the proposed Act.

To avoid the possibility of duplication with research being carried out by other Government agencies, a merger was planned between the Institutes of Experimental Biology and Medicine to form a new Institute to be called The National Institute of Arthritis and

Metabolic Disease (NIAMD) at Bethesda. A National Advisory Council on arthritis and metabolic diseases was also set up.

The combined influence and support of the Arthritis and Rheumatism Foundation and NIAMD soon started to provide the much needed funds, and American rheumatology became a fast growing American specialty. The relationship between the professional and clinical ARA and the essentially fund-raising Arthritis and Rheumatism Foundation suffered many vicissitudes. These bear a striking resemblance to those relating to the British counterparts which were the Heberden Society, the Arthritis and Rheumatism Council, and the British Rheumatism Association. In each of the associations, working for the same ultimate goal, but having started off as independent entities, rivalries developed that long delayed their amalgamation. Indeed in the UK there are still rifts between the ARC and the BRA (now Arthritis Care).

In America, talks of amalgamation between the two associations started as early as 1950, in an effort to overcome the difficulties in co-operation and co-ordination of the activities of the two organisations, thus reducing overlap and duplication.

Many members of the ARA however felt that amalgamation would weaken the professional status of their organisation of which they were so proud. During this period, between 1952 and 1953, Currier McEwen was President. In 1955 talks on amalgamation foundered and the integration committee which had been set up was dissolved. The issue remained dormant for the next five years. Finally in June 1965 the ARA merged with the Foundation, of which it became a professional section, retaining its name and independent

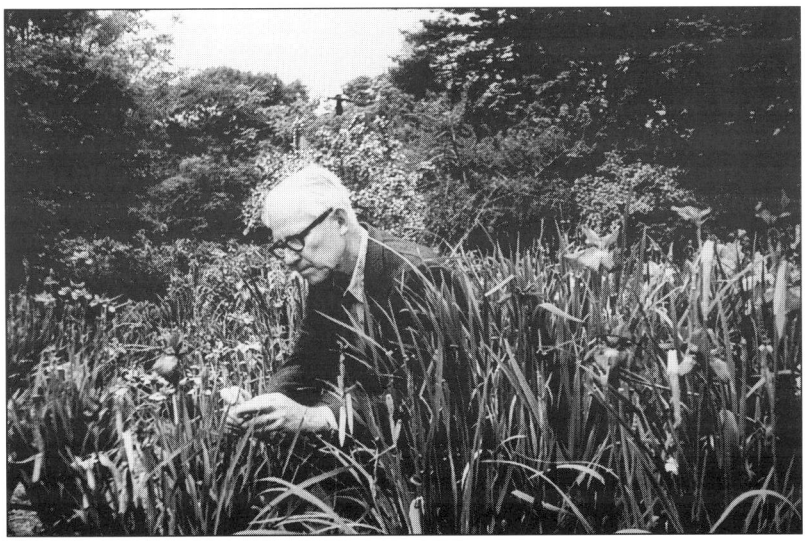

Currier McEwen (Eric Bywaters).

internal organisation. Even then the assets of the ARA were not handed over immediately to the Foundation, so that the merger could have been easily reversed if the consolidations failed. However, finally on 30 June, 1970, the remaining assets of the ARA were turned over to the Foundation and the ARA from that time onwards was known as The American Rheumatism Association section of the Arthritis Foundation. In 1976 there was a final major reorganisation of the Foundation, designed to increase efficiency and improve communications between the staff and the professional and lay volunteers.

Physiatry
In this section we shall endeavour to chronicle and compare the parallel developments of rheumatology and physical medicine (called physiatry in the USA) which were occurring across the Atlantic during the formative years.

The first and most striking difference is that, across the Atlantic, the two specialties developed independently of each other, with totally separate spheres of activity and interest. This largely eliminated overlap and conflict. Indeed, if there was any 'friction' across the Atlantic it tended to be between the orthopaedic surgeons and the physiatrists. Traditionally, orthopaedists had been accustomed to supervising and prescribing for their own patients and did not necessarily appreciate the advantage of yielding part of this responsibility to their new specialist colleagues.

In the USA, physiatry was regarded as an essentially therapeutic discipline, which provided facilities and expert advice for any disparate group who wished to make use of their services and experience. Thus it was no more concerned with rheumatological patients than with those suffering from orthopaedic, neurological, respiratory, or even dermatological conditions.

Other contrasting features existed between the American and the UK scenes; for example most American rehabilitation units had a generous supply of beds into which they could admit and supervise their own patients. In the UK, competition for limited bed space, and disputes as to the ultimate authority for the patients who occupied them, seemed to be the inevitable result of NHS stringencies.

Disputes as to whether access to the treatment departments should be 'open' or 'closed' to GPs and hospital colleagues were also a striking feature under a monopoly provider such as the NHS. However, open departments were, with occasional exceptions already noted, acceptable in America, where alternative private arrangements could be made. In addition, structured teamwork, implying a degree of joint responsibility, seems far easier to achieve under the American system than under the NHS.

Apart from the problem of therapeutic prescriptions, there was also a contentious issue concerning 'referral' policies under the NHS. Thus the consultants in charge of some departments insisted on 'primary' referral so that they should be fully involved in diagnostic and investigative procedures. They wished to receive their patients directly from the GPs. Others favoured exclusively 'secondary' referrals from hospital colleagues who would be entirely responsible for the diagnostic 'work up' before referring them. The latter system was more akin to the American system and at least it had the virtue of a clear stratification of responsibilities, and the absence of competition for scarce resources. Recently, the pattern in the UK has veered almost exclusively to the primary referral system, thereby increasing the contrast with transatlantic practice.

Typically, the American department was much more lavishly—and elegantly—equipped than its British counterpart during the period under consideration. This contrast was particularly striking in the provision of hydrotherapy facilities. Under the NHS, economic considerations tended to limit the provision and servicing of therapeutic pools and other expensive equipment to the basic minimum. In America, the 'market economy' system encouraged ever larger and better equipped amenities within their physiatry departments.

Another consideration arising from the market economy is the fact that the cost of a bed in a rehabilitation unit in the USA is considerably less than in a corresponding acute hospital bed. This naturally encourages the earlier transfer of patients for active rehabilitation than is the custom in the UK. Early treatment might represent a genuine advantage to patients suffering from certain types of disability (e.g. hemiplegics and cardiovascular rehabilitation cases). Conversely it is important to take this point into critical consideration when auditing and comparing American claims for therapeutic success and cost effectiveness with our own. It is my impression that limited facilities and consequent delays under our system result in our seeing a far higher proportion of fixed and irreversible disability than do our American colleagues. In consequence, their claims of higher success rates may be spurious, unless critically discounted against the tendency to natural remissions in the early stages of many conditions.

The history of modern American physiatry dates from the year 1890, when the American Physiotherapy Association was formed and held a meeting in New York. In 1947, immediately after World War II, specialist boards were set up with a view to defining training standards and setting examinations. In 1952 the Association was renamed The American Congress of Physical Medicine and Rehabilitation.

In 1960, a *World Directory of Physical Medicine Specialists* was produced and the American section included 500 names of whom more than 300 held specialist board accreditation.

The development of American physiatry, as in most specialties, has depended on the foresight and perseverance of certain individuals. Among those of special importance were Richard Kovacs, born 1884 who became Professor of the New York Polyclinic Medical School. He was author of a standard text book of physical medicine and of the original Year Book on the subject. He was American delegate to the 1936 International Congress on Physical Medicine held in London. Frank Krusen, born 1898, spent most of his career at the Mayo Clinic with a great interest in research and education. In 1941 he produced his first edition of his text book on physical medicine. With Howard Rusk he set up the American Board of Physical Medicine and was its first Chairman. In 1956 he instituted the American Rehabilitation Foundation Policy Group. Howard Rusk was the Director of the Rehabilitation Centre, New York Medical School and wrote both his *Text Book of Rehabilitation* in 1958, and also *Living with Disability*. He had a special interest in treatment of cardiovascular problems.

Edward Lowman moved from the Mayo Clinic to become Deputy Director of the Rehabilitation Centre, New York, under Howard Rusk. He had a special interest in the arthritic and was a very sound rheumatologist. Sydney Light worked at the Mount Sinai Hospital, New York, and also Boston and Yale. He published the *World Directory of Physical Medicine Specialists* in 1960. Richard Freyberg, the orthopaedic rheumatologist mentioned elsewhere, also did much to promote the importance of rehabilitation. Hans Kraus, Associate Professor of Physical Medicine, New York, made a special contribution to the treatment of back conditions. These are a few who contributed to the American scene in physical medicine.

Chapter 7

The Evolution and Spectrum of Rheumatic Diseases 1930-1990

'Rheumatism' is any pain occurring within a mile of a joint.
(Philip Hench)

In a period of sixty years, such as we have attempted to cover in this book, it is hardly surprising that significant changes have occurred in the patterns, incidence and severity of diseases seen in rheumatology clinics. It seems probable that the changes have been more radical in our specialty than in many others. In this chapter I shall examine some of the trends which have so greatly altered the spectrum of our clinical practices during our mutual careers.

Rheumatic fever
In the 1930s the scourge of rheumatic fever was still rampant and requiring large numbers of hospital beds. Not only was treatment protracted and demanding of resources, but the ever-present threat of permanent cardiac damage necessitated a multi-disciplinary approach to management. In the team the rheumatologist co-operated with the paediatrician, the cardiologist and, what would now be termed, the community health physician.

Contemporary Epidemiology
A recent survey gives the following statistics. The term 'arthritis' covers up to 200 different diseases. They affect:
- 20 million people
- 15,000 children
- 5% of people aged 16-44
- 41% of people aged over 65
- Over 8 million people consult their doctors every year about some form of rheumatic pain
- Every year 1½ million people attend hospital for the first time with problems relating to rheumatism and arthritis
- At least 70 million working days are lost each year through rheumatism and arthritis
- The cost of statutory services and benefits for arthritis and rheumatism approaches £1.5 billion a year.

Some reasons for the expanding spectrum
More recently, our range of interests and clinical responsibilities has greatly increased. Several factors have contributed to the need

for the contemporary rheumatologist to receive a full training in general medicine before practising as a specialist. Some of the developments underlying the widening range of rheumatological 'catchment' are definable.

Immunopathology and Rheumatology
There has been an evolving, and increasingly sophisticated appreciation that disorders of immunological tolerance underly many of the systemic rheumatic diseases. This, together with new concepts of the pathology of connective tissue in general and the collagen and micro-vascular systems in particular, have enlarged not only our understanding, but also the clinical 'catchment' which we could include under the umbrella term of 'rheumatology'.

Endocrine and Metabolic Diseases
The same consideration applies to the rapidly expanding field of metabolic bone disease and calcium metabolism, as it became evident that many endocrine and metabolic disorders can present with obscure 'rheumatic' symptoms.

Methods of Investigation
The equally rapid advance in methods of investigation during the period has enabled earlier recognition of many diseases, and the more accurate categorisation of others. This in turn has resulted in some major revisions of our concepts of the natural history and prognosis of certain diseases. For example, until about twenty years ago, a diagnosis of systemic lupus erythematosus was tantamount to a death sentence. Nowadays, when the diagnosis is frequently made at a very early stage of the disease, it is recognised that there are milder variants which are compatible with long-term survival with minimal suffering.

'New' and Newly Interpreted Diseases
Many apparently 'new' diseases have been described during our period. Some of these are undoubtedly the result of new clinical and neuro-physiological observations enabling a reinterpretation of previously described syndromes. A few appear to represent entirely new diseases. We could cite as examples of these two groups:

The appreciation of the relationship between chondrocalcinosis, pyrophosphate arthropathy and pseudo-gout in 1963.

The concept of 'compression neuropathies' in general, and the carpal tunnel compression syndrome in particular, which has so greatly modified the management of conditions such as acroparaesthesiae, and sciatica, which were previously regarded as having a 'rheumatic' basis. It was not until 1934 that Mixter and Barr[1] described herniations of the intervertebral disc as the basis of many nerve root compression syndromes.

Polymyalgia rheumatica (see p 22) is now regarded as a common cause of rheumatism in the elderly. Previously it was probably confused with carcinomatosis and 'fibromyalgia', which remains an obscure and under-researched area of rheumatology. However, the recognition of its association with arteritis, especially of the temporal arteries leading to potential blindness, has emphasised its greater significance as has its excellent response to corticosteroids.

'Enteropathic arthritis' is another concept linking several gastro-intestinal diseases with inflammatory joint disease, and possibly yielding hints as to their common aetiologies. Certainly this important association had not been generally recognised before the 1960s.

A few genuinely 'new' diseases do seem to have arisen, and a search through old text books is unlikely to reveal, either by name or description, any condition resembling, for example, relapsing polychondritis,[2] which was first described in 1960. Or the so-called 'overlap syndromes' such as 'mixed connective tissue disease' described by Sharpe in 1972[3] and 'eosinophilic fasciitis', described by Shulman.[4] Even more novel is the polyarthritis described about four years ago under the eponymous title of 'Lyme disease'.[5] This is a tick-transmitted spirochaetal infection described in 1975 following a commendable piece of medical detective work on an epidemic which started in the small town of Lyme in Connecticut, and which appears to be spreading.

Non-Rheumatic Diseases Presenting with Skeletal Pains

Because rheumatism clinics have the facilities for treating musculo-skeletal pains by physical methods, there is a tendency to refer to them a wide range of medical and surgical conditions which have nothing in common except for skeletal pain. Much of this clinical material is unsorted and lacks a satisfactory diagnosis. Apart from acting as a diagnostician, the rheumatologist, if only for the convenience of his patient, frequently has to accept responsibility for the total care of such patients. For example, the differentiation of osteoporosis from the various forms of osteomalacia, and the treatment of both forms of bone pain would be accepted within his province, as would the management of Paget's disease with calcitonin, diphosphonates or mithramycin.

Unusual diseases of immigrant populations have added a further interpretive interest to the responsibilities of rheumatological clinics with a greatly extended microbiological spectrum and a required essential knowledge of cultural and dietetic habits which might contribute to ill health.

Eclectic Case Loads

The merging of the disciplines of 'rheumatology', physical medicine and rehabilitation, and the simultaneous training of rheumatologists in all three disciplines has, of necessity expanded the clinical load of contemporary departments of rheumatology. It is true that some specialised 'centres of excellence' persist in which the range of conditions are restricted to systemic rheumatic diseases. But in general, district hospitals run eclectic programmes in which, for example, a case of 'tennis elbow' may be followed by one with a life-threatening collagen-vascular disorder.

Medical Orthopaedics
In addition, over-worked orthopaedic departments tend to delegate to rheumatology departments much of their commitment which has been described as 'medical orthopaedics'. Since this may include the primary management of backache, the influx of such patients may well outnumber those suffering from specifically 'rheumatic' conditions.

Another 'para-orthopaedic' commitment happily undertaken by departments of rheumatology since the early 1950s has been the intra- and peri-articular injections of corticosteroids, which has proved to be very sparing of physiotherapy time in suitable cases.

Prophylactic, salvage and replacement surgery
A more direct association with orthopaedic colleagues has arisen because of the exciting developments in corrective and prophylactic 'rheumatological' surgery. The forward planning of a surgical programme for a patient suffering from polyarthritis must take account not only of medical, but also of social and domestic considerations. It has therefore become the practice of most rheumatology departments to organise regular combined clinics, in which surgeons, physicians, physio- (and occupational) therapists, together with social workers, meet and confer about their patients' needs.

Sports medicine
The current interest in the specialty of sports medicine and soft tissue trauma has also resulted in a closer association between rheumatologists and their colleagues. Many sports medicine clinics are located, if only for logistical reasons, within departments of rheumatology, creating a further diversification of interests.

Rehabilitation
The commitment of rheumatology departments to the many facets of rehabilitation medicine has proved contentious—as has been pointed out earlier. In future, it is probable that rehabilitation will become a totally separate discipline, situated in the near vicinity of a specialised rheumatic unit. In the meanwhile, financial and

practical constraints ordain that much of the work of rehabilitation is carried out within the orbit of departments of rheumatology. As an example of the diversity of interest in which this may result, several departments have organised specialised cardiac rehabilitation units within their confines.

Electrodiagnosis

It may cause surprise to future generations to learn that the disciplines of electrodiagnosis were largely developed in physical medicine departments. The explanation is that some of the therapeutic machines, such as faradic and galvanic stimulators, were used to carry out the crude testing of neuromuscular integrity. The early electromyograph machines were usually situated in departments of physiotherapy and these were followed by machines which measured nerve conduction velocities. It seems likely that future generations of registrars will be spared at least this part of their training, as specialist neurophysiologists become available to develop and take over these important disciplines.

References

1 Mixter WJ, Barr JS. Rupture of intervertebral disc with involvement of spinal canal. *New Eng J Med* 1934; **211**: 210.
2 Mitchet JM Jr, McKenna CH, Outhero HS, O'Fallon WM. Relapsing polychondritis. Survival and predictive role of early disease manifestations. *Ann Int Med* 1986; **104**: 74.
3 Sharpe GC, Irwin WS, Tan EM, Gould RG, Holman HR. Mixed C-T Disease. An apparently distinct rheumatic disease syndrome associated with a specific antibody to extractable nuclear antigen (ENA). *Am J Med* 1972; **52**: 148.
4 Shulman LE. Diffuse fasciitis with eosinophilia: a new syndrome? *Trans Assoc Am Phys* 1975; **88**: 70.
5 Steere AC, Malavista SE, Snydman DR *et al.* Lyme arthritis. An epidemic of oligo-articular arthritis in children and adults in three Connecticut communities. *Arth Rheum* 1977; **20**: 7.

Chapter 8

Evolution and Spectrum of Drug Therapy

Pre-war to the 1950s
In our chapter on 'The Clinical Picture in the 1930s' we outlined the problems and horrors of the rheumatic diseases in the pre-war era. It would now be helpful to outline further the development of the drug treatment which has revolutionised their outlook.

As previously stated, rheumatic fever in children and recurrences, often with mitral stenosis, filled most beds that could be spared for rheumatology. Salicylate was the only palliative remedy. The discovery of the aetiological significance of the *Streptococcus viridans* by Lancefield in 1940[1] and then its susceptibility to antibiotics—the sulphonamides[2] and later to penicillin—associated with better hygiene and less overcrowding, rang the knell for this condition.

For rheumatoid arthritis, the salicylates and aspirin were the only treatment and this often resulted in peptic ulceration and haematemesis. In the early 1930s, the Forestiers at Aix les Bains[3] noted the resemblance of some of the patients to those suffering from tuberculosis and therefore started to use gold injections. High and prolonged medication, disregarding early signs of toxicity, resulted in renal damage and rashes proceeding to exfoliative dermatitis and blood dyscrasias, but many showed some improvement in their arthritis.

Stanley Davidson, then Professor of Medicine at Edinburgh, switched his interest from anaemia to the problem. He was not impressed and did much to instigate the ERC multi-centre research trial of 200 cases in 1960,[4] the first trial of its kind and magnitude, undertaken on the general assumption that it would debunk the treatment. It was not a fair trial, weighted against it being its rigidity, which denied any clinical flexibility. Yet it came out directly in favour of the gold-treated cases to the surprise of three-quarters of the participants. Myocrisin (sodium aurothiomalate) was given, with a miniscule dosage as control. Only 5% developed toxic symptoms necessitating withdrawal from the trial and the remainder received benefit for about a year after discontinuing the gold. Gold was then the only 'disease modifying drug' that affected the disease itself.

The treatment of gout with colchicine dates back to the fifth century when it was known as hermadactyl. To produce an early effect, the dosage had to be pushed up till it produced diarrhoea and nausea. Cinchophen was also used, but here there was a real danger of producing acute yellow atrophy of the liver. Control of the acute attack with colchicine has now been largely superseded by the use of phenylbutazone (Butazolidin) or indomethacin (Indocid).

Then in 1937 Jennings[5] demonstrated the uricosuric effect of the salicylates, but they frequently produced some gastric disturbance and dizziness. In 1951 Talbott[6] showed a similar and greater effect on the uric acid excretion using Benemid (probenecid) and then in 1958 sulphinpyrazone (Anturan) proved even more effective.[7] Probenecid was originally developed as a 'sparer' of penicillin by inhibiting the excretion by the renal tubules and this lead to the discovery that it also inhibited the urates. The problem with the uricosurics however was that they tended to clog up the kidneys and to produce calculi, but they remained the prime treatment, till the breakthrough of the discovery of xanthine oxidase inhibition by allopurinol (Zyloprim) in 1959.[8] This reduced the production of uric acid instead of just washing it away.

References
1 Lancefield RC. Haemolytic streptococci. *Harvey Lectures* 1940-41; **36**: 251.
2 Coburn AF, Moore LV. The Sulphonamides. *J Clin Invest* 1939; **18**: 147.
3 Forestier J. Gold treatment in rheumatoid arthritis. *Rev Rhum Mal Osteoartic* 1935; **2**: 472.
4 ERC Trial of Gold. Chloroquinine in rheumatoid arthritis. *Ann Rheum Dis* 1960; **9**: 95.
5 Jennings GH. Use of salicylates or uricosurics in gout. *Rep Chr Rheum Dis* 1937; **3**: 106.
6 Talbott JH. Use of benemid in gout. *Proc Inst Med Chir* 1951; **18**: 383.
7 Hobbs HE, Calnan GS. Use of sulphur pyrazone in gout. *Lancet* 1958; **i**: 1207.
8 Hobbs HE. Allopurinol and xanthine oxidase inhibition in gout. *Lancet* 1959; **ii**: 478.

1949-1990

Corticosteroids
Occasionally, rheumatologists use the acronym 'BC/AC' when discussing the history of developments in the therapy of the rheumatic diseases. The 'pivot' year referred to is 1949, when the potential complete suppression of rheumatic inflammation by the use of corticosteroids (and corticotrophin), was first demonstrated. Previously, treatment had been directed at the suppression of symptoms, as opposed to inflammatory pathology.

Initially heralded as the long-awaited panacea in the management of rheumatic diseases, it was not long before the appreciation of unacceptable and seemingly inevitable side-effects precluded the use of corticosteroids except in certain well defined, and frequently very

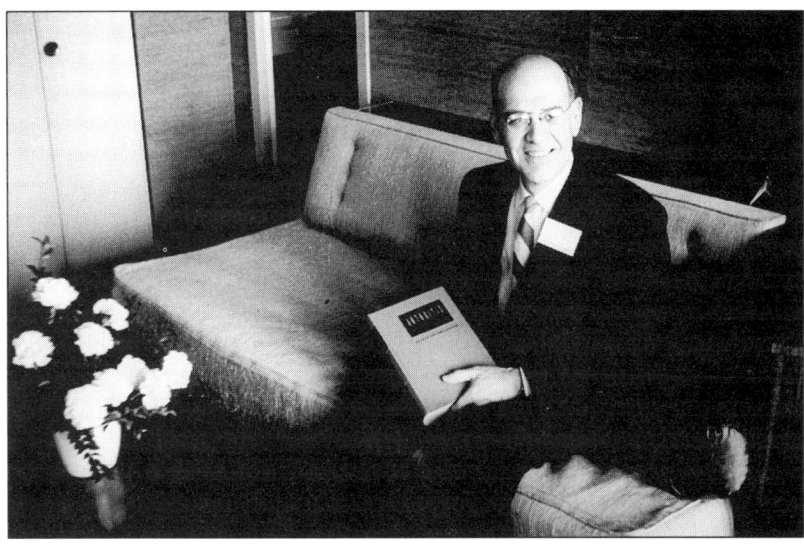

Joseph Hollander (Eric Bywaters).

severe diseases. In the light of subsequent history, it seems that the pendulum of prejudice against steroids swung excessively. Indeed it was not until 1955, as supplies improved and prednisolone became available, that a balanced opinion developed as to their clinical indications and modes of use.

Less controversial, and probably just as important in practical terms, has been the local use of corticosteroids by their injection directly into joints or painful areas of soft tissue, largely piloted by Hollander and his group in Philadelphia.[1] Curiously this potential for relatively safe corticosteroid therapy was initially not appreciated because cortisone itself is inactive if administered locally. Pending the development of a technique for converting a ketone to a hydroxyl radical at the 17 position of the steroid nucleus, creating hydrocortisone (and all its subsequent analogues), all steroid treatment had to be administered systemically with its attendant and inevitable profile of unwanted effects.

Non-Steroidal Anti-inflammatory Drugs
Meanwhile there began a frantic and frustrating search for safer corticosteroid analogues. Later the spotlight of pharmacological research concentrated on the considerable difficulties of mass production of active steroids. Paralleling this, and just as intensive, was the search for non-steroidal 'anti-rheumatic' drugs which might be used either on their own, or in combination with smaller doses of steroids, in which case they were sometimes known as 'steroid sparers'.

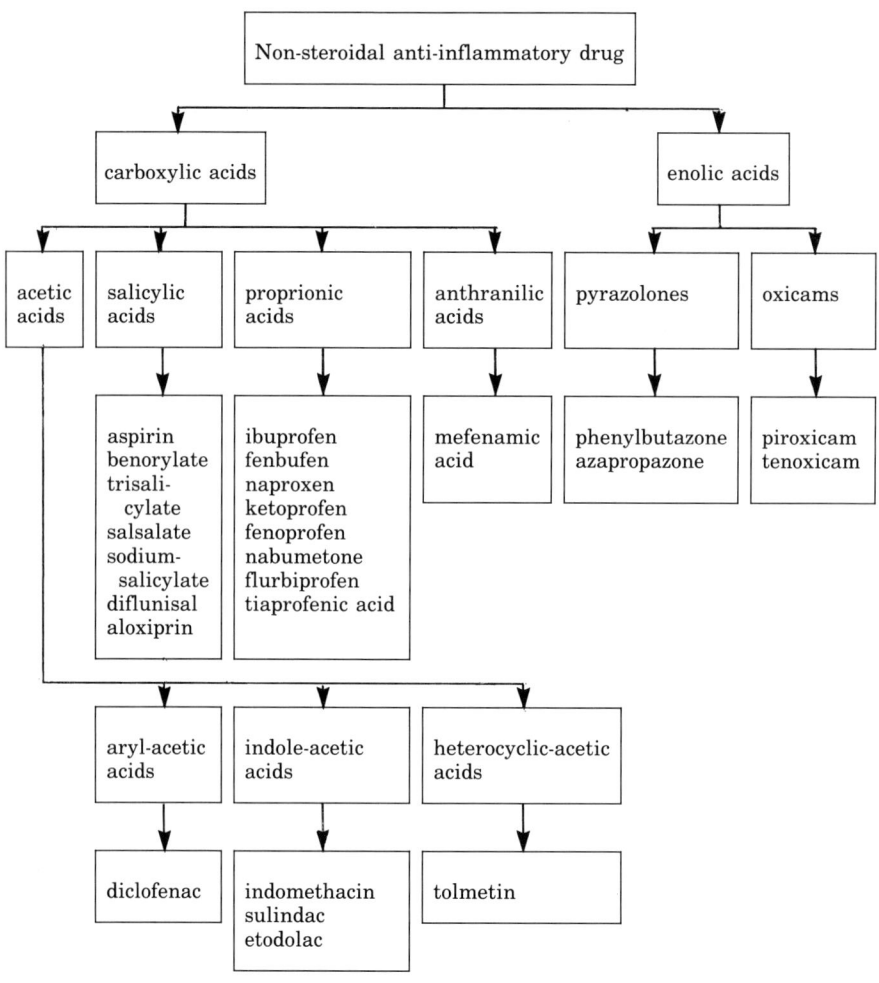

The progeny of some of the more commonly used non-steroidal anti-inflammatory drugs

Phenylbutazones

The discovery of the first of these 'non-steroidal anti-inflammatory drugs' (NSAIDs)—phenylbutazone—seemingly occurred by serendipity. The Swiss pharmaceutical company Geigy wished to market an injectable preparation of the powerful analgesic amidopyrin. The most appropriate solvent proved to be phenylbutazone. They marketed the solution under the trade name of 'Irgapyrin'. However, they encountered considerable sales resistance, notably from British physicians, who felt that amidopyrin, whether in injectable or oral formulation, was an unacceptable drug to use in the treatment of chronic pain. This was because of its notorious reputation for producing agranulocytosis.

Approximately one year after the introduction of Irgapyrin, Messrs Geigy announced that following comparative trials they had discovered, much to their surprise, that the solvent had a beneficial anti-inflammatory activity on its own account and unrelated to the amidopyrin. They proposed to deplete the active principle entirely and to market the solvent separately under the trade name of Butazolidin!

Subsequent clinical trials indicated that it was consistently effective in the treatment of acute gout and ankylosing spondylitis, but somewhat less predictable in controlling the synovitis of rheumatoid arthritis. For good measure, it was also found to be very effective in the management of phlebo-thrombosis and, finally, the veterinary fraternity discovered that 'Bute' made race horses (presumably 'rheumatic' sufferers!) run much faster!

Phenylbutazone and its later analogue oxyphenylbutazone were prodigiously prescribed between the early 1950s and the beginning of this decade, when the media chose to launch a virulent attack on its safety record.

Apart from some relatively rare and usually reversible side-effects (such as oedema, which can cause encephalopathy), there were reported approximately five hundred cases of irreversible and therefore fatal aplastic anaemia. Resulting from the detrimental publicity, the drug was withdrawn from general circulation and now only prescribed from hospital pharmacies for the treatment of ankylosing spondylitis and acute gout.

Whilst not denying its occasional potential for causing serious haematological toxicity and an unfortunate, but manageable, propensity for retaining sodium it would seem, on a statistical basis, that the risk to any individual was extremely slender, and that panic may have deprived us of a drug which was capable of giving considerable relief and comfort when appropriately prescribed.

Indomethacin and later NSAIDs
In the twenty-eight years since phenylbutazone was released, an ever increasing flood of NSAID preparations have been marketed, their bewildering profusion indicating that the 'ideal' drug, in terms of consistency, potency and safety, still eludes us. The immediate successor to phenylbutazone was indomethacin, which was based on an indole-acetic nucleus and which appears to have stood the test of time as well as the large number of its successors. In truth, all of these NSAID preparations are capricious and unpredictable in their actions, so that the clinician is forced into a 'trial and error' situation when selecting one or other preparation for an individual patient.

There appears to be a common principle underlying the versatile pharmaceutical search for new preparations, namely the inhibition of one or more of the enzyme systems which mediate inflammation at the periphery. Thus prostaglandins not only act as mediators in their own right but also accentuate the inflammatory response to other mediators such as kinins and histamine.

Despite their considerable structural differences, virtually all the NSAID preparations do inhibit prostaglandin synthetase, and part of their anti-inflammatory potency presumably depends on this action.

However, there are other enzyme systems, such as the lipoxygenase system, which NSAIDs do not inhibit and this may be the explanation of their therapeutic inconsistency and unpredictability. Unfortunately, the inhibition of prostaglandin synthesis is not selective for areas of inflammation, and in situations—such as the gastric mucosa—where prostaglandins exert a *protective* effect, inhibition may be undesirable, leading to mucosal damage and ulceration.

It is for this reason that many patients find the entire group of NSAIDs unacceptable in terms of dyspepsia which can progress to serious gastrotoxicity. Attempts are being made to overcome this problem by the use of what are called 'pro' drugs, which do not become activated until they have safely passed through the stomach and duodenum. Other attempts to mitigate this problem have been to add supplementary H_2 antagonists to the regime, and, more recently supplementary prostaglandins have been combined with the NSAID formulation.

The final verdict on the NSAID era remains to be written. Certainly we may hope for future improvements both in terms of safety and effectiveness. Meanwhile, there can be few rheumatologists who would not regard them as a modest but important advance in terms of the management of their patients. Physiotherapists have also had cause to bless them, when pain relief has eased their task of maintaining mobility and preventing the development of contractures.

Disease Modifying Drugs
The ultimate therapeutic objective in the management of a disease must surely be to eradicate—as opposed to suppress—the underlying pathology. Rheumatologists so far have not achieved this 'dream', but certainly not from want of trying.

Several of the more important developments have occurred as a result of astute clinicians, who have made observations on their rheumatoid patients who were being treated for quite different conditions. The observations by Forestier on the rheumatological benefits of the injections of gold salts intended as treatment for their associated phthisis is perhaps the classical example of this type of 'lateral thinking'.

Anti-malarial drugs in rheumatology
Another good example, was the observation by Francis Page when, in the course of his national service, he was designated as a

dermatologist and was posted to the tropics. He noted that patients suffering from discoid lupus erythematosus, tended to improve when exposed to the Mepacrin tablets which had recently been introduced by the army for routine malaria prophylaxis.

Despite the fundamental differences between discoid and systemic lupus erythematosus, it was not long before physicians were reporting improvements in patients suffering from the latter disease when treated with chloroquine (and subsequently hydroxychloroquine), which soon became the favoured anti-malarial drugs, as they were less toxic than the original Mepacrin. From here it was but a short intellectual jump to suggest a trial of anti-malarial drugs for the treatment of rheumatoid arthritis. Anti-malarial therapy (as previously described) soon had an established place in the management of rheumatoid disease. Its benefits, whilst seldom spectacular, can usually be achieved in the absence of serious side effects.[2]

D Penicillamine
Penicillamine was originally used as a chelating agent in the treatment of heavy metal poisoning. Paradoxically, it was even tried in America in cases of gold poisoning in patients receiving chrysotherapy, but was subsequently abandoned in favour of dimercapto-propanol (BAL). It remains however the standard treatment for the chelation of copper in cases of hepatolenticular degeneration (Wilson's disease). It was also used in cases of cystinuria to prevent the formation of cystine stones.

It was noted by Jaffe in 1963 in the USA that it was capable of dissociating the components of the rheumatoid factor complex.[3] In those days it was felt that the rheumatoid factor might play a pathogenetic role in the development of the disease and as a corollary, the breakdown of the associated immunological complex might provide a logical approach to the therapy.

Once again, the logic may have proved to be spurious, but careful clinical assessment over the next few years vindicated Jaffe. Penicillamine has proved to be approximately as potent as gold as a therapeutic agent. It is also approximately as toxic—albeit with a different range of side-effects. There is a characteristic latent interval before it produces its acknowledged beneficial effects. Whilst it is in no sense a therapeutic 'breakthrough', it constitutes a useful 'disease modifying' therapy. Some patients find it more beneficial and acceptable than chrysotherapy, but unfortunately this preference is capricious and largely unpredictable in an individual sufferer.

Sulphasalazine
In the 1940s Nana Svartz became interested in a possible relationship between gastro-intestinal flora and polyarthritis.

Her observations were originally made on patients suffering from ulcerative colitis who were treated with sulphasalazine (a combination of the recently discovered antibiotic sulphapyridine and a salicylate 5-amino salicylic acid). She observed unexpected improvements in the associated polyarthritis suffered by some of the patients and later claimed significant benefit in patients suffering from classical rheumatoid polyarthritis.

However, despite her pre-eminence as a senior Professor of Medicine at the Kariolinska Institute in Stockholm, this form of therapy did not become established at the time. In 1978 a British physician (McConkey) re-appraised and reported favourably on its effectiveness in the treatment of rheumatoid and similar types of polyarthritis.[4] It would now seem that sulphasalazine has a small, but secure, niche in rheumatological therapy.

Local use of anti-proliferative drugs
Rheumatoid granulation tissue is proliferative and erosive. As such it bears certain resemblances to the invasive pathology of cancer. This led, inevitably, to trials of drugs which appeared to be able to inhibit the proliferation of cancerous tissue, either by a direct cytotoxic effect, or by interfering with the immunological processes underlying the proliferative pathology.

It was during the mid 1950s that the systemic, and the intra-articular use of various nitrogen mustards was advocated by Jimenez-Diaz[5] from Barcelona. They enjoyed a short vogue in the UK, which was limited largely by their painful and other unpleasant side-effects. In the Heinola Rheumatism Centre in Finland, the use of osmic acid intra-articularly became a standard therapy, but this also produced extremely painful reactions which limited its popularity. More recently, enthusiastic claims have been made for what has been termed a 'chemical synovectomy' by the intra-articular injection of a beta emitting radio-active isotope of yttrium.[6] This form of therapy is not painful and appears to be associated with few and trivial unwanted effects. When combined with a simultaneous injection of an anti-inflammatory corticosteroid, the benefit seems to be enhanced and speeded.

Immuno-suppression
Chlorambucil, azathioprin and cyclophosphamide have all been advocated and subjected to careful clinical trials in the last twenty-five years. Unfortunately their undoubted usefulness in controlling intractable rheumatoid inflammation has to be balanced against the unpleasant toxic effects and because they may cause carcinogenesis.

Currently, the folic acid antagonist, methotrexate, is enjoying a resurgence of popularity in the UK and the USA. Originally found very effective in the management of psoriasis, it was soon noted to benefit the associated arthritis which frequently afflicts psoriatic patients. Its routine use in the treatment of rheumatoid disease has been inhibited in the past by its reputation for hepatotoxicity and the necessary precaution of repeated liver biopsies. However, current thinking suggests that the risks, in the rather low dosage regimes recommended, have been exaggerated and that with routine blood monitoring, liver biopsies may not be required.

More recent developments in the management of gout
The potent suppressive effects of both steroid and non-steroidal anti-inflammatory drugs in acute attacks of gout has dramatically improved and shortened the management of the 'agonies' of the acute gouty attack. However, it is in the interval management of the hyperuricaemia underlying the disease that developments have been most exciting.

We have noted the unsatisfactory use of high doses of salicylate as a uricosuric: probenecid was originally intended as a 'sparer' of penicillin in the early days when supplies of this were very short. Excretion of penicillin by the renal tubule was inhibited. By the same token, it inhibits the reabsorption of urates as they pass through the tubules resulting in 'uricosuria'. It has the additional virtue of once a day dosage.

Sulphinpyrazone is related to phenylbutazone, but it has a weaker anti-inflammatory action. It does have a significant uricosuric effect. Because it needed to be administered three times a day, and also because it was occasionally gastrotoxic, it never attained wide usage in the UK.

Xanthine oxidase inhibition
As previously mentioned, the major breakthrough in the management of gout and its complications occurred when Allopurinol became available.[7] Allopurinol is an isomer of hypoxanthine and acts by competing with the enzyme xanthine oxidase which is essential for the conversion of hypoxanthine and xanthine into uric acid.

Once again, this invaluable clinical advance arose on the basis of serendipity. Allopurinol was originally discovered for the therapy of leukaemia. It was to be used in association with the cytotoxic drug 6-mercaptopurine to prevent the oxidation of the active drug to an inactive metabolite.

Allopurinol is relatively non-toxic and is administered on a long-term basis to limit hyperuricaemia. It is so effective and consistent in its effect that it is possible to 'titrate' the dosage against serum levels of uric acid until this reaches a level at which the patient is unlikely to suffer further attacks of acute gout. It is also possible to 'leach' sodium biurate from tophaceous deposits thus significantly reducing their size.

References
1 Hollander JL, Jessar RA, Restifo RA, et al. *Arth Rheum* 1961; **4**: 422.
2 Page F. Treatment of lupus erythematosus with Mepacrine. *Lancet* 1951; **ii**: 755.
3 Jaffe IA. Penicillamine: an anti-rheumatoid drug. *Am J Med* 1963; **75**: 63.
4 McConkey B, Amos RS, Durham S, Forster PCG, Hubbal S, Walsh L. Sulphasalazine in RA. *Br Med J* 1980; **280**: 442.
5 Jimenéz-Diaz C. Treatment of dysreaction diseases with nitrogen mustard. *Am Rheum Dis* 1951; **10**: 144.
6 Wingfield J, Gumpel JM. An evaluation of repeat intra-articular injections of Yttriam 90 colloids in persistent synovitis of knee. *Ann Rheum Dis* 1979; **38**: 145-7.
7 Rundles RW, Metz EN, Silberman HR. Allopurinol in the treatment of gout. *Ann Int Med* 1966; **64**: 229.

Chapter 9

The Evolution of Rehabilitation

In previous sections we have traced some of the developments that have occurred during the last fifty years concerning the understanding and practical management of the rheumatic group of diseases. In so doing we have made several references to developments in the field of 'rehabilitation' during the same period.

A 'panoramic' view of these developments reveals philosophical and practical changes in attitudes and practice which, in their own way, are every bit as startling as those in the strictly rheumatological fields and they deserve to be chronicled separately.

Without doubt, the main impetus for change emanated from the armed services during both, but especially the second, world wars. Manpower shortages dictated that physical and psychological casualties needed to be returned to 'battle fitness' as rapidly as possible and, as a corollary, maximum co-operation and motivation by the patients was also essential. In order to encourage this attitude, rehabilitation was presented in the form of a personal challenge to the injured and one of the most successful techniques took the form of competitive games in which mental distraction of the patient from his own sufferings played an important role, whilst tending to minimise those introspective neuroses, which were so prevalent in the 1914-18 conflict.

Another major conceptual development from the services was the appreciation that rehabilitation usually involves team work covering many different disciplines. It was in the armed services that such diverse approaches could be welded into 'tailor-made' programmes appropriate to the specific requirements of each casualty. Such team work of necessity required a leader to co-ordinate the team, and from such leaders emanated the vanguard of the post-war rehabilitation specialists. Names such as Frank Howitt, representing the army, and EE O'Malley in the RAF spring to mind in this context. In the case of the RAF, there was an additional 'drive' from the powerful orthopaedic duet of Sir Reginald Watson-Jones, who was the civilian consultant and Sir Henry Osmond-Clarke, the senior orthopaedic consultant within the service. As a result of their combined enthusiasms and skills, the RAF developed highly sophisticated methods of returning injured personnel to active combat in minimum time. Such centres of excellence as the one at Chessington and its complementary centre for officers at Hedley Court, long outlasted the war period and were the exemplars of many of the civilian centres set up in the NHS after 1948. During the war the high cost of training and shortage of pilots gave the RAF financial priority in the setting up and equipping of such rehabilitation centres.

Whilst it remains true that locomotor disability still constitutes the heaviest clinical load of patients requiring rehabilitation (approximately a third of the total), it soon became evident that the philosophy and techniques developed in relation to locomotor problems could be well adapted to the management of many other types of disability.

Another disease group, for example, which places very heavy demands on civilian rehabilitation centres arises from patients who have suffered 'strokes' and other chronic neurological conditions. Such conditions inevitably respond slowly and recovery is rarely complete and therefore, in every instance, a careful 'cost/potential benefit' analysis should be carried out before committing skilled staff to the slow and frequently frustrating process of rehabilitation.

In such cost/benefit analyses, several factors are of paramount importance. The first is the actual, and also the 'potential' motivation of the disabled. In the past, patients have been unfairly castigated for lack of progress and lack of motivation, without appreciating the indisputable fact that organic brain damage frequently results in the destruction of those psychological centres from which initiative and motivation emanate.

It is essential to evaluate this factor *before* making a commitment to long-term treatment. Indeed in the long run it is kinder both to the patient and the therapist so to do. Selection should also, as far as is possible, be uninfluenced by sentiment, tragic as some of the resulting decisions may appear at the time.

An important factor in the evaluation of rehabilitation is the stage of the illness at which it is commenced. This may depend on pragmatic economic factors etc. Thus, for example, in most centres in the USA, the comparative cost of hospitalisation in an 'acute' bed, and residence in a rehabilitation unit greatly favours the latter. As a result, rehabilitation in the USA tends to start at a significantly earlier stage than is possible within the limited resources for intensive treatment in the NHS.

It could be argued that the availability of early treatment is an unmitigated advantage for a patient. However, bearing in mind the immense difficulty of predicting the body's capacity for spontaneous recovery, especially following seeming neurological 'catastrophes', it seems likely that some of the effort expended on early cases may be wasted, as the patient would probably have achieved the same improvement unaided. Certainly this factor should be taken into consideration when comparing the effectiveness of rehabilitation techniques between one community and another.

Another post-war development in the philosophy of rehabilitation was the acceptance of *realistic*, as opposed to *optimal*, goals of achievement. These should always relate to the patient's dignity and associated independence, but they should also take account of the type of work of which he is intrinsically capable (albeit with special training in some instances) and also his, or her, domestic and financial circumstances. The concept of sheltered employment has been an important and successful development in this context. The law directing that three per cent of all labour forces must be registered as disabled has not had such a great impact, because of the ease with which it can be evaded.

Because it was appreciated that most rehabilitation needs to be intensive and programmed between active and rest periods, the tendency has been for specialist centres to become residential. This, whilst adding to the cost, introduces compensatory psychological advantages—namely, camaraderie and competitiveness.

The competitive aspect and the realisation that personal problems are not unique and are usually matched by others, who have equal or more serious physical and psychological battles to fight, may be a considerable bonus. Unfortunately cost may rule out this ideal. The Peto Centre in Budapest treats congenital diplegic children all day, five days per week for years. It would be economically impossible to provide this for every child who might get marginal benefit from such therapy. Therefore, careful pre-selection of candidates is essential.

Another interesting post-war development has been the adaptation of engineering and electronic principles to the aid of the disabled. The ingenuity involved has been prodigious and complex, but the importance, so far as rehabilitation is concerned, is the acceptance that rehabilitation is, and should be, a multi-disciplinary specialty. Centres for evaluation of apparatus have become commonplace in this context.

While the friction between rheumatology and rehabilitation have now largely disappeared, the two specialties will not become synonymous. The field of rehabilitation is now so wide that a physician rheumatologist would not have the time or incentive to become closely involved. However, as an exception to this trend, in 1977 the Royal National Hospital for Rheumatic Diseases, Bath, was designated a centre of excellence for teaching and research in both rheumatology and rehabilitation and Dr Tony Clarke was appointed as both Director of Rehabilitation and Consultant in Rheumatology.

Meanwhile, the pattern of rehabilitation has altered and is now largely devoted to neurology, including cardiovascular incidents, and traumatology. At specialist centres, apart from teaching, much time is devoted to assessment of new techniques and investigation of home aids which reduce the need for in-patient care.

In rheumatology, despite its high incidence, relatively few osteoarthritics are admitted except following surgery. A bed count at the Bath hospital in 1989 showed an admission list of approximately 9% for rehabilitation, especially selected as suitable after accidents, strokes and a few with disseminated sclerosis. The remainder consisted of about 70% cases of complicated polyarthritics and connective tissue disorders, 15% spondylitics, 4% for the investigation of osteoporosis and only about 2% for osteoarthrosis.

Specialised rehabilitation
We have discussed some of the historical reasons for the close associations between the disciplines of rheumatology and rehabilitation, and also the recent 'breakaway' trends. In this section, we shall attempt to peer prophetically into the future of the rehabilitation services.

It seems inevitable that rehabilitation will eventually become a separate discipline with its own training programme. Pending a much needed rebuilding programme however, departments of rehabilitation will probably retain their traditional 'geographical' locations within departments of physiotherapy.

The concepts and achievements of 'rehabilitation' have recently broadened to an extent that its economic and humanitarian benefits to the community are easy to demonstrate. As a result it has proved attractive to successive Ministers of Health who, hopefully, will continue to support its development within the NHS, including the creation of more centres of excellence.

Because the primary objective of rehabilitation is to return as many sick patients, as soon as possible, to their natural habitats, a costly long stay in an institution should be avoided if possible. By contrast, the main justification for residential rehabilitation centres is to evaluate disability and, having trained the patient in the best ways of overcoming it, to return him to the community. The philosophy guiding all rehabilitation planning should relate to the independence of, and the restoration of dignity to, the disabled.

Viewed in these terms, the expansion of the specialty will certainly breach the relatively narrow confines of orthopaedics, neurology and rheumatology, where it all started.

As an example, many cardiologists are already enthusiastic that patients benefit from programmes of structured rehabilitation following coronary infarcts and also following cardiac surgery. Such programmes include progressive exercising, monitored by sophisticated measurements and appropriate psychosomatic re-education.

Carried out within the protected confines of a Rehabilitation Centre it helps to restore confidence and persuade patients that they are capable of resuming active and useful lives when they are discharged.

The prevailing policy of closing long-stay mental hospital beds has recently provoked our psychiatric colleagues to develop necessarily specialised rehabilitation programmes, designed to ease the return of the mentally sick to the world outside.

In fact, so many varied specialties, faced with the bed shortages and high costs of acute hospital care, are devising their own programmes of rehabilitation, that it would be inappropriate to list and discuss them individually.

Sophisticated refinements in domestic rehabilitation cannot be separated from advances in non-medical technology, notably in the field of electronics. Thus, the wizardry by which so many domestic activities can be operated from an electronic keyboard may revolutionise the independence and life-style of the most severely disabled patients. For example, a quadraplegic can be taught to operate such a device from his wheelchair by means of a light pointer clasped between his lips.

Even greater electronic wizardry will be required within the current attempts to produce a computerised muscle stimulator which would assist paraplegics to walk by mimicking the extremely complex, sequential pattern of muscle contraction that is required for normal gait. Early prototypes of such machines already exist in research laboratories and it would seem that the concepts of 'bionic' or 'robotic' man should no longer be regarded as exclusively within the province of science fiction.

Such measures are inevitably extremely costly and must be planned with discretion, as indeed should all aspects of rehabilitation programmes. It is important that physicians, politicians and administrators alike should distinguish between those measures designed as humanitarian contributions and those designed to be cost effective. Either stratagem, or a judicious mixture of both, may be justifiable, depending on the context of the case. Effective strategic planning, however, demands that the 'paymaster' understands the motivations behind the appeals for support in order to maintain a balance between competing 'empires'.

Audit is now much under debate. Clinical audit must be beneficial, but financial audit is usually painful when planning rehabilitation and rheumatology services.

Using Diagnosis Related Groups (DRG) from this point of view could be misleading. Too short hospitalisation can temporarily save money, but in the long term cost more. In one study reducing hospitalisation from 22 to 13 days, 22% more patients were discharged to less costly nursing homes, but 33% compared with 9% remained in a nursing home after a year.

In addition the application of DRG is not easy in rheumatology. For instance a psoriatic arthropathy could be categorised as psoriasis or polyarthritis with quite different effect on the audit. The interpretation of financial audit can therefore be difficult to interpret and even open to abuse.

Chapter 10

The Evolution and Process of Fusion

This personal anecdote is intended to illustrate the type of rivalry which existed between the two specialist groups in the post war era.

Following my training as a rheumatologist and my research fellowship in New York, it became evident that in order to return to the NHS training ladder, it would be necessary to obtain a training post as a senior registrar, preferably in a teaching hospital. There appeared to be no possibility of achieving this on an exclusively rheumatological unit for which there was, as yet, no official establishment. I was fortunate therefore, in 1953, to obtain a senior registrar's post in Dr William Tegner's physical medicine department at the London Hospital.

Effectively, the work and clinical experience was identical to that of a rheumatology department, but for traditional and personal reasons Tegner's loyalties remained with physical medicine which meant that I had now crossed 'the great divide'.

The passage however was not a smooth one and I was aware that I had to present a very low profile until, hopefully with the passage of time, I became acceptable to my new colleagues.

Within a few weeks of arriving at the London Hospital, a clinical conference was arranged to take place with our Belgian colleagues in Ostend and Bruges. It had been privately organised by a senior member of the British Association of Physical Medicine who had Belgian connections.

The meeting was pleasant and friendly until the moment of departure, by bus, from our hotel, to the channel port.

I then became aware of some agitated discussion between our 'leader' and a reception clerk from the hotel who announced that one of our number had not settled his indebtedness for 'extras' spent in the hotel. Being convinced that I had incurred no such extras I was disinterested in the proceedings until my room number was read out.

On enquiry, it seems that, according to my habit at that time, I had left my shoes in the corridor and that they had been cleaned for which a charge (which I well remember, was the equivalent of one shilling and eight pence—approximately 8p—had, unknown to me, been placed on my account.

Not only was I publicly upbraided on the bus for 'letting the side down' but I received an official reprimand later from a member of the committee. He told me that the matter would be reported to the President (who, at that moment was none other than Lord Horder).

I don't believe that he took a very serious view of my misdemeanour, and apart from a feeling of humiliation and probable stain on my reputation the incident was forgotten.

However trivial this episode may appear on recounting it, I was convinced at the time, and remain so, that it symbolised the tension and resentment felt by one wing of the specialty against the other. In this case it concerned the infiltration into their allocation of training posts. Such jealousy might seem inconceivable in today's happy symbiosis but it was a recurring and important feature of the development of our specialty in my early days.

Recent developments
Gradually, both rheumatology and rehabilitation became recognised as respectable specialties, and the battle between them eventually came to an end. Many physicians at special centres remained pure rheumatologists. At smaller general hospitals there were general physicians with a special interest in rheumatology, in other places the consultant was responsible for rheumatology clinics and physical medicine departments.

In previous chapters we have told of the divisions and consequent friction that existed between the specialties of rheumatology, physical medicine and rehabilitation. The process of 'fusion', which forms the natural conclusion of our story, was slow and painful.

Despite recognition by many 'senior brethren' (and none more so than our senior author GDK) of both specialties, an increasingly ludicrous and untenable situation developed. The main impetus for fusion emanated from our younger members.

Probably, the irresistible impetus for fusion arose from the largely common study programmes required of its trainees leading to a genuine camaraderie and sympathy between the registrars irrespective of their sponsorship or specific aspirations. It became increasingly evident that, apart from a few ultra specialist departments, the clinical spectra and responsibilities of either specialty were remarkably similar and overlapping. Indeed, clinical case loads tended to reflect the special interests of the consultant in charge more accurately than the departmental labels ascribed by the hospital appointment committees.

And yet, despite these overwhelming sentiments, the process of political fusion was an extremely prolonged and tortuous process. It started unofficially in 1963, when a working group of registrars representing both disciplines held informal discussions. Despite the goodwill of all those concerned, their efforts proved abortive and were abandoned after a few months.

Towards the end of the 1960s, Michael Mason in his capacity of President of the Section of Physical Medicine of the Royal Society of Medicine, tried unsuccessfully to add the word Rheumatism to the title of the section. As his section secretary during his year of

THE HEBERDEN SOCIETY

ANNUAL DINNER

1972. Dr. A. C. ALLISON, M.Sc., M.A., D.Phil.
1973. Professor Mu Dr St. SITAJ, Dr. Sc.
1974. Professor D. A. WILLOUGHBY, Ph.D., M.R.C.Path., F.I.Biol.
1975. Dr. LAWRENCE E. SHULMAN, M.D., Ph.D.
1976. Dr. HELEN MUIR, M.A., D.Phil., D.Sc.
1977. Dr. BARBARA M. ANSELL, F.R.C.P.
1978. Dr. J. T. DINGLE, D.Sc., Ph.D.
1979. Professor J. E. SEEGMILLER, M.D.
1980. Professor S. D. KRANE, M.D.
1981. Professor ROY M. ACHESON, D.M., F.F.C.M., F.R.C.P.
1982. Dr. DANIEL J. McCARTY, M.D.
1983. Professor J. J. VAN ROOD

HONORARY MEMBERS

Dr. R. G. ABERCROMBIE
M. C. G. ANDREWS, C.B.E.
Professor Sir MELVILLE ARNOTT, T.D.
Professor J. DE BLECOURT
Professor A. BONI
The Rt. Hon. The Lord BRAIN, F.R.S.
Dr. C. W. BUCKLEY
Dr. W. BYAM, O.B.E.
Professor E. G. L. BYWATERS, C.B.E.
Professor Sir ERNST CHAIN
Professor Sir JOHN CHARNLEY, C.B.E.
The Rt. Hon. The Lord COHEN
Professor F. COSTE
Professor Sir STANLEY DAVIDSON
Professor J. DECKER
Dr. M. M. DESAI
Professor J. I. R. DUTHIE
A. G. T. FISHER, F.R.C.S.
Dr. J. FORESTIER
Professor Sir FRANCIS FRASER
Dr. L. E. GLYNN
Dr. M. GORDON, C.M.G., C.B.E., F.R.S.
Professor J. GOSLINGS
Dr. F. D. HART
Dr. C. B. HEALD, C.B.E.
Dr. P. S. HENCH
Dr. A. HILL
S. L. HIGGS, F.R.C.S.
The Rt. Hon. The Lord HORDER, G.C.V.O.
Sir W. WILSON JAMESON, G.B.E., K.C.B.
Professor J. H. KELLGREN
Professor E. C. KENDALL
Dr. G. D. KERSLEY, O.B.E.
Professor F. LENOCH
Dr. E. LEWIS-FANING
The Rt. Hon. The Lord MORAN, M.C.
Dr. K. MUIRDEN
Dr. D. MURRAY LYON
Dr. S. NELSON
Dr. M. B. RAY, D.S.O., O.B.E.
The Lord RICHARDSON, M.V.O.
Dr. R. G. ROBINSON, O.B.E.
Dr. OSWALD SAVAGE, O.B.E.
Professor HANS SELYE
Professor S. DE SEZE
Dr. W. S. TEGNER
Prof. Sir RONALD TUNBRIDGE, O.B.E.
Lord WEBB-JOHNSON, K.C.V.O., C.B.E., D.S.O.
Professor Sir LIONEL WHITBY, C.V.O., M.C.
Professor L. J. WITTS, C.B.E.
Professor M. ZIFF
Professor N. ZVAIFLER

GLAZIERS HALL
LONDON BRIDGE

ON

THURSDAY, 10th NOVEMBER, 1983

President:
PROFESSOR D. A. BREWERTON, F.R.C.P.

MENU

Prawn and Apple Cocktail

—:—

Onion and Anchovy Tartlets

—:—

Duck Breasts en Croute
with Orange Sauce
Potatoes

—:—

Profiteroles with Whipped Cream

—:—

Coffee

—:—

Pouilly Fume 1982
Mouton Cadet 1979/80
Port or Brandy

TOASTS

THE QUEEN

THE GUESTS
Proposed by THE PRESIDENT

Reply by THE RT. HON. LORD GRIMOND

BRITISH RHEUMATOLOGY
Proposed by PROFESSOR J. VAN ROOD

THE NEW SOCIETY
Proposed by DR. J. T. SCOTT, F.R.C.P.

The last Heberden Society Annual Dinner and Foundation Dinner of the British Society of Rheumatology, 1983.

office, I became well aware of the unreasonable passions evoked by this attempt, which was doomed to failure at the time, although it was this section which a few years later proved to be the vanguard of change by becoming officially the Section of Rheumatology and Rehabilitation in 1974.

The Diploma of Physical Medicine examination set up originally in 1948 was also abandoned at about this time (1974) in favour of a Diploma of Rehabilitation Medicine which was instituted a few years later.

In 1970 the Association of Physical Medicine decided to change its official title to the British Association of Rheumatology and Rehabilitation (BARR) and in August of that year their official journal, *The Annals of Physical Medicine*, appeared with its cautious change of title to *Rheumatology and Physical Medicine*. This changed to *Rheumatology and Rehabilitation* in February 1973 and it finally became *The British Journal of Rheumatology* in 1984 at the time of the final merger.

Meanwhile, very slowly, and ponderously initially, discussions took place between the hierarchies of the Heberden Society and BARR and these led in January 1984, following complicated postal ballots, to the dissolution of both Societies in order to create the one official Society called the 'British Society for Rheumatology' which now satisfactorily represents the clinical, political and research interests of our broad spectrum specialty, now internationally known under the single name of 'rheumatology'. The *British Journal of Rheumatology* has become the official organ of the Society, although the prestigious *Annals of the Rheumatic Diseases* continues to prosper independently. The name of William Heberden continues to be honoured via the annual Heberden Oration and Heberden Rounds. In addition the official library of the Society is still housed in the Heberden Room at the Royal College of Physicians.

Chapter 11

Epilogue

We have now completed our survey of the remarkable developments that have occurred in the fields of rheumatology and allied specialties over the last sixty years. It is expedient to view the acknowledged disappointments and frustrations of our dreams of a therapeutic 'breakthrough', within the time spans of our mutual professional careers, in the context of the 'Cinderella' status of our specialties at the start of our story.

The story we have attempted to tell of two feuding groups who failed, for nearly fifty years, to appreciate their complementary interests and ultimate common destiny, together with their tortured efforts to overcome their mutual antipathies, is by no means unique in medical circles. An analogous situation arose when the British Tuberculosis Association expressed their wider interests by renaming themselves the British Thoracic Society before they finally amalgamated with the general chest physicians as The British Thoracic Association. Without doubt similar situations will arise in the future as new specialisms develop and wish to establish their own identities.

Perhaps there are lessons to be learned. Certainly our specialty would by now be in an even stronger position had we presented a united front at an earlier date and certainly those of us who participated in the events recorded would have been spared much unnecessary anguish and tribulation!

Rheumatology and rehabilitation are now living together in happy symbiosis with some overlap, but each recognised as a reputable clinical, teaching and research entity.

It seems permissible to end on an optimistic note by recording the excellent recent recruitment of high calibre, clinical and scientific trainees into our chosen field. If only because of this, we are blessed by a feeling of confidence that our subject will continue to prosper.

Perhaps the epitaph of our generation should read: 'we fought a hard battle and laid strong foundations!'

Biographies

In this section there is a series of very short biographies of many of those who contributed most to the history of rheumatology and rehabilitation. To avoid repetition the following recognised abbreviations are used.

Empire Rheumatism Council—ERC, later the Arthritis and Rheumatism Council—ARC
La Ligue Contre le Rhumatism—La Ligue
The International League against Rheumatism—ILAR
The European League against Rheumatism—EULAR
Pan American League Against Rheumatism—PANLAR
SE Asian, Pacific and Australasian League—SEAPAL
The British League against Rheumatism—BLAR
The British Association of Physical Medicine—BAPM, which became in 1970 The British Association of Rheumatology and Rehabilitation—BARR, and which amalgamated with the Heberden Society in 1984 to become The British Society for Rheumatology—BSR
The British Rheumatism Association—BRA, which became Arthritis Care
The Peto Place Red Cross Clinic—Peto Place, which became The Arthur Stanley Institute of the Middlesex Hospital

Roy Acheson DM MD ScD FRCP FFCM
From Dublin he moved to Oxford to qualify in 1957. He held the first Chair in Community Medicine at Cambridge. His oration was on Epidemiology and the Arthritides.

Robert Cairns Aitken MD FRCP Psych DPM
Qualified in 1957 at Glasgow. After a Senior Lectureship in Psychology at Edinburgh, he became Professor in Rehabilitation Studies at Edinburgh University.

Anthony Allison MSc BM DPhil
Qualified at Oxford in 1952 after working in South Africa. He worked for 20 years with the MRC and then moved to the California Institute of Technology. His oration was on Tolerance and Autoimmunity.

Michael Andrews CBE
Born 1918. Secretary of SSAFA before becoming Secretary General of the ARC in 1956. Here he quietly and self effacingly, did more on the organisational side to bring about its financial and administrative success than would have seemed possible.

Barbara Ansell CBE MD FRCP
Qualified at Birmingham in 1946. She joined Eric Bywaters at Taplow and then Hammersmith and later became Head of the Division of Rheumatology and Clinical Research at Northwick Park. She has been an Orator and President of the Heberden Society. Her main interest has always been paediatric rheumatology in which field she is world famous.

Wm Melville Arnott, Sir William Kt TD MD FRCP FRCPath FRSE
Qualified at Edinburgh in 1931. He became Professor of Medicine at Birmingham and was a member of the UGC and MRC. He was a founder member of the ERC and an Honorary Member of the Heberden Society.

Francis Bach MD DPhys Med
Qualified in 1925 Oxford and St Bartholomew's Hospital, London. He was a Consultant in Physical Medicine to the EMS during the war. He was the medical mainstay of the BRA in its early years.

Paul Bacon MD FRCP
Qualified Cambridge and St Bartholomew's Hospital, London in 1963. After a consultancy at the RNHRD at Bath, he became Professor of Rheumatology at Birmingham.

George Baehr
Emanated from Friburg and Vienna, but emigrated to New York, where he originally worked in the Mount Sinai Hospital in New York and became Professor of Medicine at the College of Physicians and Surgeons, Columbia. He later became Medical Director of the US Public Health Service. He had a primary interest in infections of neoplastic disease, but will be best remembered for his work on the pathology of connective tissue disease, in which subject he published definitive papers with Drs Klemperer and Pollack.

John Ball BSC MD FRCP (Path)
Qualified in 1941 at Manchester, where he became Professor of Osteo-Articular Pathology. He did some early work on electron microscopy and then on enthesopathy and the importance of bone ligament functions, especially in spondylitis. He has been President and Orator of the Heberden Society.

H Wykham Balme MD FRCP
Qualified 1943 Cambridge and St Bartholomew's Hospital, London. Director of the Department of Rheumatology, St Bartholomew's Hospital. Cattlin Research Fellow.

Pedro Barcelo
Dr Pedro Barcelo who led the field in rheumatology in Spain in the 1960s was a President of both ILAR and EULAR.

Colin Barnes MD FRCP BSc
Qualified at the London Hospital in 1961 where he became Consultant in Rheumatology. He did gallant work as Chairman of the ARC and was President of BLAR and now of EULAR.

Walter Bauer BS MD FACP
Qualified in 1922 at the University of Michigan. He became Jacksonian Professor of Medicine at the Massachusetts General Hospital and Harvard. At first interested in metabolic studies of bone disease, he became involved in research in rheumatoid arthritis, on which he gave his Heberden Oration.

Philippe Bauwens
Qualified at St Thomas's Hospital, London, in 1924 where he took charge of the Electrotherapy Department. In this subject he became an international authority. He became a Founder Member and the first Secretary of the BAPM.

David R Blake MRCP
Qualified at Sheffield in 1974. After registrarships at Bath and Birmingham, he is now Professor of Rheumatology at the London Hospital.

Jan de Blecourt MD
Qualified at Leyden in 1941 and became Director of Rheumatology at Groningen. He played a large part in international rheumatology as Vice President of EULAR. In particular he was the founder of the Committee of Social and Community Agencies which brought into the League representatives of the physiotherapists and other bodies dealing with rheumatic suffering.

AC Boyle MD FRCP DPhys Med
Qualified at the Middlesex Hospital in 1941 and went into the army as a Physical Medicine Specialist. He later obtained his MD, FRCP, DPhys Med and became Director of the Department of Rheumatology at the Middlesex. He was the first Chairman of the reconstituted BLAR Scientific Committee in 1972.

Walter Russell Brain, the Rt Hon the Lord Brain DM PRCP FRS DSc DCL LLD
Qualified at the London Hospital in 1922. His main career was in Neurology at the Hospital for Nervous Diseases and the London Hospital. Knighted 1952, he became Baron in 1962, while President of the Royal College of Physicians. He gave his oration to the Heberden Society on Spondylosis.

J Van Breeman MD
Was born 1873 in Holland and was largely responsible for the formation of the Society for Physical Therapy in 1905, the International Society for Medical Hydrology and La Ligue Contre le Rhumatism. A further history of his contributions to rheumatology will be found in the text.

Barry Bresnigham MD FRCP FRCPI
Qualified 1968 at University College, Dublin. Consultant in Rheumatology St Vincent Hospital, Dublin. He has been a Heberden Roundsman and Gravis Lecturer. He is a Member of British Association of Physicians. He was capped several times for Ireland.

Derrick Brewerton BSc MD FRCP DPhys Med
Qualified in 1947 in Montreal. He later became Consultant at the Royal National Orthopaedic Hospital and then at the Westminster with a Personal Chair in Rheumatology. At first involved in the care of the physically handicapped, he then did important work in the genetic field on HLA B27 in ankylosing spondylitis. He was the last President of the Heberden Society before it was amalgamated with BARR to form BSR.

Knud Brochner-Mortensen MD
Qualified MD at Copenhagen where he became Professor of Medicine. He gave the Heberden Oration on Gout, which was one of his main interests.

Charles Buckley MD FRCP
Born 1874. Qualified 1916 at St Mary's, London. He was Mayor of Buxton in 1924 and Senior Physician to the Devonshire Hospital, Buxton. He was a member of the Royal Colleges Committee and then of the ERC and edited the *Reports* of both organisations. He was a President of the Heberden Society. He did much to bring Spa medicine into line with academic Internal Medicine.

Joseph Bunim MD ScD FACP
Was born in Russia and qualified MD in New York in 1930. After research on haemolytic streptococci in rheumatic disease at Yale, he returned to Bellevue. In 1952 he established the Institute of Arthritis and Metabolic Diseases at Bethesda. He was President of the American Rheumatism Association. His oration was on Sjögrens syndrome.

Barnes Burt MD
Qualified at University College Hospital, London in 1902. He became a Spa Physician at Buxton and then moved to the Royal National Hospital for Rheumatic Diseases (then the Mineral Water Hospital) at Bath. Here he played a part in making it a true centre for rheumatology.

Hugh Burt MD MRCP
Was the son of Barnes Burt. He qualified Cambridge and University College Hospital, London in 1937. In 1942 he became one of the original army team of Physical Medicine specialists. He was later a Secretary of the ARC and won a Heberden Prize.

Eric Bywaters CBE MD FRCP
Qualified at the Middlesex in 1933. After valuable research work, he was appointed to the British Post-Graduate Medical School at Hammersmith and later to the Canadian Red Cross Hospital, Taplow. He became the second Professor in Rheumatology in the country in 1958. He was a President and Orator of the Heberden Society and did much to build up its library of which he was Librarian for twenty years. He was chairman of the Scientific Advisory Committee of the ARC for ten years.

Andrei Calin MD FRCP
Qualified at Cambridge in 1968 before spending some years in America and then joining the Royal National Hospital for Rheumatic Diseases at Bath where he was Chairman for its 250th Anniversary.

Norman Capener FRCS
Qualified at St Bartholomew's Hospital, London, in 1922 and then moved to the Princess Elizabeth Hospital at Exeter, where he became the uncrowned king of orthopaedics, which he considered also covered arthritis.

Ernst Chain Sir Ernst Kt D Phil PhD FRS
Was a joint discoverer of penicillin for which he shared a Nobel Prize and he also discovered D-penicillamine. He took his PhD in Berlin 1930 and fled to Cambridge to do research in biochemistry. After a spell in Rome he returned to become Professor of Biochemistry at Imperial College, London. He was elected a Heberden Honorary Member for his contribution to therapeutics.

Marcella Anne Chamberlain BSc DCh FRCP
Qualified at Guys in 1964. After a Senior Registrarship at the Middlesex Hospital in Rheumatology and Rehabilitation, she became Professor of Rehabilitation Medicine at Leeds.

John Charnley Sir John Kt CBE DSc FRCS FRS
Qualified at Manchester in 1935. He was the first to tackle the engineering principles of joints, to provide the first reliable arthrodesis of the knee and later arthroplasty of the hip.

During the war he was Consultant in Orthopaedics to the RAF and developed the adjustable Thomas splint. He became Professor of Orthopaedic Surgery at Manchester and did much to develop the Wrightington Hospital Centre at Wigan.

Anthony K Clarke BSc MD FRCP
Qualified at the London Hospital in 1968. He joined the staff of the Royal National Hospital at Bath as the first joint Director of the Centre of Excellence for Teaching and Research into Rehabilitation and Consultant in Rheumatology.

Vincent Coates MC MD FRCP
Qualified at Cambridge in 1920. He joined the staff of the Royal Mineral Water Hospital (RNHRD) at Bath where he did much to bring it into the twentieth century. He was on the first committee of La Ligue and was an International Rugby player.

Henry Cohen, Rt Hon the Lord CH DL JP MD FRCP DSc LLD
Born 1900 he qualified at Liverpool where he became Professor of Medicine in 1934. He was President of the BMA, the GMC, the RSM, the Association of Physicians and a Harvean Orator. After chairing the Ministry of Health Committee on Rheumatology, he became President and then Orator of the Heberden Society. He was knighted in 1949 and became Baron in 1956.

Frank Cooksey CBE MD FRCP DPhys Med
Qualified King's College Hospital in 1929. He became Director of the Physical Medicine Department there. He did much to organise rehabilitation in the EMS during the war, for which he was awarded the CBE. He was a President of the BAPM.

Will Copeman CBE TD JP MD FRCP
Born 1900 he qualified St Thomas's Hospital 1925. After an interest in paediatrics at the West London Hospital, he launched into rheumatology. He was Medical Secretary and later Chairman of the ERC; a Founder Member, President and Orator of the Heberden Society; a Vice-President of the Royal College of Physicians; and Master of the Apothecaries. He received the OBE in 1945 and CBE in 1964. He developed the Heberden Library and was a keen medical historian. His constant fight was to put rheumatology on the map as a respectable specialty.

Florent Coste MD
Qualified 1921 in Paris having already received the Croix de Guerre in World War I. In 1948 he became the first Professor in Rheumatology at the Hôpital Cochin and with Forestier firmly divided arthritis into inflammatory and degenerative types. He was a President of La Ligue (1957-61) and gave a Heberden Round in 1950.

Stephen Crane MD FACP
Trained at the Massachusetts General Hospital in 1951 and later became Professor of Medicine at Harvard. He worked especially on

metabolic bone disease and gave his Oration on Cell Biology of the Rheumatoid Synovial Lesion.

Warren Crowe DM
Qualified at Oxford and St Mary's Hospital London, in 1902. He was Director of the Charterhouse Rheumatism Institute and Consultant in vaccine treatment at the Home for Incurables.

Harry Currey M Med FRCP DA
He qualified Cape Town in 1950 and joined the London Hospital becoming Professor of Rheumatology there and Director of the ARC Bone and Joint Research Unit in 1973. He was a President of the Heberden Society and gave his Round on Rheumatological Renal Disease.

James Cyriax MD
Qualified Cambridge and St Thomas's Hospital in 1929. He was manipulative surgeon to the Charterhouse Clinic and became Director of the Physiotherapy Department at St Thomas's Hospital, where he followed in the steps of JB Mennell in the study of the value of manipulation.

Stanley Davidson, Sir Stanley Kt MD FRCP PRCP Ed FRCS Ed
He qualified in 1919 after service in World War I. He became Regius Professor at Aberdeen before returning to Edinburgh. He was President of the Association of Physicians and a Heberden Roundsman. He promoted rheumatology in Scotland and was largely responsible for Ian Duthie's taking up this specialty.

John Decker MD FACP
Graduated at Columbia University in 1951. He did much of his research into clinical rheumatology, especially on lupus, at Bethesda and was voted an Honorary member of the Heberden Society.

Madhusudan Desai MD
Pioneered rheumatology in India from his HQ in Bombay. He was President of the Association of Physicians and of Cardiologists of India. He was Founder President of the Indian Rheumatism Association, a President of SEAPAL and an Honorary member of the Heberden Society.

Paul Dieppe MD FRCP
Qualified at St Bartholomew's Hospital, London, in 1970 and in 1987 became Professor of Rheumatology in Bristol. Has taken a special interest in degenerative joint disease.

John Dingle PhD DSc
From a research assistantship at the RNHRD at Bath, he joined Dame Honor Fells at the Strangeways at Cambridge where he

became Deputy Director. Having a special interest in the effect of lysosomes on connective tissue, he gave his Oration on the Control of Joint Damage.

Allan St John Dixon MD FRCP
Qualified at Guy's in 1945. After working in China and New Zealand, he returned to the Postgraduate Hospital at Hammersmith and Taplow. Thence he came to the Royal National Hospital for Rheumatic Diseases at Bath and became a visiting Professor at Bath University. He was Founder Chairman of the Back Pain Society and of the National Ankylosing Spondylitis Society and Adviser in Rheumatology to the DHSS. He was a President of the Heberden Society.

Ian John Duthie FRCP
He qualified Edinburgh in 1935 and was chosen by Professor Sir Stanley Davidson to take a lead in rheumatology in Scotland. He became a Professor in 1968 of Edinburgh University and was a President of the Heberden Society. He did valuable work on splintage in arthritis and the anaemia of rheumatoid disease. He was Specialist in Physical Medicine, RAMC.

Ernest Lewis Fanning PhD DSc
Was one time Secretary to the MRC and became the statistician to the ERC and did much to establish clinical trials on a statistical basis. He was made an Honorary member of the Heberden Society. From London he moved to the Welsh National School of Medicine.

Dame Honor Fell DBE PhD DSc FRS
Came from Edinburgh. She later became the Director of the Strangeways Research Laboratory at Cambridge, where she did important work on tissue culture. Her Heberden Oration was on The Role of Biological Membranes on Skeletal Reactions.

Ernest Fletcher MD FRCP
Qualified Cambridge and St Bartholomew's Hospital, London, in 1918. He joined the Consultant staff of the Royal Free and the Arthur Stanley Institute. He was a President and the first Orator of the Heberden Society.

Jacques Forestier MD
Was son of Henri Forestier and was co-founder of La Ligue. In World War I he was given the *Croix de Guerre* and *Legion d'Honneur* and afterwards became an Olympic athlete. He then pioneered the rheumatology clinic at the Hôpital Cochin in Paris and did important work on radio-opaque oils before returning to Aix les Bain. There he instituted gold treatment in rheumatoid arthritis and in his later

years described ankylosing intervertebral hyperostosis. He was a mainstay of La Ligue of which he became President and he was a Heberden Orator.

R Fortescue Fox MD FRCP
Qualified at the London Hospital in 1882. He was a leading spirit in the foundation of the International Society for Medical Hydrology, La Ligue Contre le Rhumatism and the Peto Place Clinic. A further history of his contributions to rheumatology will be found in the text.

Francis Fraser, Sir Francis MD FRCP Ed FRCP
Qualified Cambridge and Edinburgh in 1910. He came to St Bartholomew's Hospital, London, as Professor of Medicine, was Director General in Medicine to the EMS and then became Director of the Post-Graduate Medical Federation at Hammersmith.

Michael Freeman MD FRCS
Qualified Cambridge and the London Hospital 1957. Fellow of the British Orthopaedic Association. Consultant in Orthopaedic Surgery, the London Hospital. First to use a Condylar knee prosthesis and to research other prostheses.

Richard Freyberg MD
Qualified in 1930 at the University of Michigan. Originally an orthopaedist he became a rheumatologist and moved to New York as Professor of Medicine at Cornell. He was President of the American Rheumatism Association, RANLAR and was a founder of the Arthritis Foundation.

Dugald Gardner MSc MG FRCP Ed FRCP Path
He first went to Cambridge for his BA and then to Edinburgh where he qualified in 1948. He was the first Director of the Kennedy Institute. His Heberden Oration was on the microscopic technology used in the study of cartilage.

John Glyn MD FRCP DPhys Med
Qualified Cambridge and Middlesex Hospital in 1947. He was President of the RSM Section of Physical Medicine and Rheumatology. Has taken a special interest in the problems of steroid medication apart from his specialisation in both rheumatology and rehabilitation. Senior Assistant Physician to Arthur Stanley Institute and later consultant to St Charles Hospital which merged with the St Mary's Hospital Group. Consultant at Prince of Wales General Hospital, Tottenham.

Leonard Glynn MD FRCP FRCPath
Qualified at University College Hospital, London, in 1934. He then specialised in pathology, working at the MRC unit at Taplow and

became Director of the Kennedy Institute. He was a Founder Fellow of the Royal College of Pathologists and a Heberden President and Orator. He was an authority on auto-immunity in rheumatic disease.

Mervyn Gordon CMG CBE DM FRS
Qualified at St Bartholomew's in 1898 where as a pathologist he worked on viruses, Hodgkin's Disease and differentiation of streptococci. He was a founder and later honorary member of the Heberden Society. He opened a research laboratory at the Mineral Water Hospital (RNHRD) at Bath in 1921 to study protein shock and streptococcal complement fixation tests.

Johan Hans Gosling MD
Qualified at Leiden in 1927 and became head of the new Department of Rheumatology there in 1939. He did much, with Van Breemen and Forestier, to found rheumatology as we know it today with a multidisciplinary approach. He was a leader in Leiden City Council and Church Council.

Rodney Grahame MD FRCP
Qualified at Guy's Hospital, London in 1955. He was President of the BSR and a Research Fellow at the Kennedy Institute. He is a Consultant and Professor in Clinical Rheumatology at Guy's. He is President of BLAR.

Guttmann, Sir Ludwig CBE FRS MD FRCP
Took his MD in Freiburg in 1924 and came as a refugee to UK qualifying in 1939. He established the rehabilitation unit for paraplegics and spinal injuries at Stoke Mandeville in 1950 and later the International Olympics for the disabled.

'Frankie' Dudley Hart MD FRCP
Qualified at the Westminster Hospital in 1933. After war service as Lt Col he returned to take charge of rheumatology at the Westminster. He was a President of the Heberden Society. He is best known for his wide interest in clinical rheumatology.

Ian David Haslock MD
Qualified in Edinburgh and then moved to a Consultancy in Rheumatology at Teeside and also a Research Fellowship to the Department of Engineering at Newcastle. He became President of the BSR.

Clifford Hawkins MD FRCP
Qualified at Guy's in 1939. His special interests were gastro-enterology and rheumatology which he pursued at Birmingham. He was a President of the Heberden Society.

CB Heald CBE MD FRCP
Born 1892. Qualified St Bartholomew's, London 1910. He later joined the staff of Royal Free and Middlesex Hospitals. He became a President of the Heberden Society and was awarded the CBE in 1919.

Phil Hench MD MS ScD LLD FACP (Hon)
He qualified at Pittsburgh in 1916 and went to the University of Minnesota where he obtained his MD. In 1926 he became Consultant in Rheumatology at the Mayo Clinic. He started to preach the importance of rheumatology before World War II, when he was promoted to the rank of Colonel. He became Editor of the *Annual Rheumatism Reviews* and President of the Arthritis and Rheumatism Association. He then became involved in the isolation of Compound E for which he and Kendall obtained the Nobel Prize as described elsewhere. He gave a Heberden Oration on the Reversibility of Rheumatoid Arthritis. He died in 1965.

Sydney Higgs FRCS
Born 1892. Qualified at St Bartholomew's, London 1927. After service in the RN in World War I, he became an Orthopaedic Surgeon at St Bartholomew's Hospital, London. He was a President of the British Orthopaedic Association and the only Orthopaedist to become a President of the Heberden Society.

Alan Hill MC FRCP
Qualified at Edinburgh in 1939. In 1952 he became Consultant Rheumatologist to Stoke Mandeville Hospital and Regional Adviser in Rheumatology to the Oxford Region. He was a President of the Heberden Society and Chairman of the League meeting, when it was held at Brighton. He was interested in serological changes in inflammation in rheumatic fever and in rheumatoid arthritis. He also organised many therapeutic trials.

Austin Bradford Hill, Sir Austin KBE PhD FRS DSc MD FRCP
Took his PhD in economics at University College in 1926. He joined the MRC and became Professor of Statistics to the School of Hygiene and Tropical Medicine. His Heberden Oration was on Reflections on Controlled Trials. He will perhaps best be remembered as he who first brought true statistics into medical research.

Leslie Hill MD FRCP
Qualified at Birmingham and the London Hospital in 1924. He became Consultant to the Royal Devonshire Hospital at Buxton and then moved to the RNHRD at Bath. He gave the Lumlean Lecture at the College of Physicians on Systemic Lupus.

Joseph Lee Hollander MD
Qualified at Cornell University in 1935. He was consultant to Surgeon General US Dept of the Army. Chief of the Section of Arthritis, University Hospital, Philadelphia. Emeritus Professor of the Medical School, University of Pennsylvania. Specialised in clinical and basic research on joint physiology and the immunopathogenesis of rheumatoid arthritis. Introduced technique of intra-articular corticosteroid therapy. Succeeded to the editorship of Comroe's *Arthritis*.

Lennox Holt MD DCH FRCP
Qualified at Manchester in 1957. After a spell at Hammersmith he returned to Manchester in charge of the Rheumatology Research Trust and as Consultant to the Royal Infirmary, Manchester and the Royal Devonshire Hospital at Harrogate. He was an ARC Research Fellow and Heberden Roundsman.

Thomas Horder, Rt Hon The Lord Cr CVO Kt MD FRCP
Born 1871. With an entrance scholarship he qualified at St Bartholomew's in 1894 and became full physician there in 1921. He was Physician to Edward Prince of Wales, George VI and Queen Elizabeth and received a Knighthood in 1918, KCVO 1925, Baron 1933, GCVO 1938. He was the first Chairman of the ERC Scientific Committee, first President of the BAPM, a President and Orator of the Heberden Society and a Harvean Orator. He perhaps did more than anyone to start both rheumatology and rehabilitation on the road to respectability.

Frank Howitt CVO MD FRCP
Born 1896. Was in the Royal Flying Corps in World War I. He qualified at Guy's 1923. He then became Director of the Physical Medicine Department at the Royal Free Hospital. He was appointed a CVO for attendance on George V in 1929. He was a Founder Member of the Peto Place British Red Cross Society Clinic and was the first President of the Heberden Society. He was a Master of the Apothecaries. Promoted Brigadier he headed the team of Army Physical Medicine Specialists in World War II.

Graham Hughes MD FRCP
He qualified at the London Hospital in 1964 with prizes in medicine, surgery and pathology and became Head of the Rheumatology Unit at Hammersmith and Consultant in Rheumatology at St Thomas's Hospital. He has become an authority on connective tissue diseases, especially on systemic lupus erythematosus on which he gave the Heberden Round.

Edward Huskisson BSc MD FRCP
Qualified at St Bartholomew's in 1964. He became Consultant in Rheumatology at St Bartholomew's and at the King Edward VII Hospital, taking a special interest in drug therapy. He was a Heberden Roundsman.

Wilson Jamieson, Sir Wilson GCB KCB MD FRCP DPh
Qualified in 1909 at Aberdeen. He became Professor in Public Health in London and then Chief Medical Officer at the Ministry of Health. He did a great deal to promote rheumatology in the earliest years and was made an Honorary Member of the Heberden Society.

Malcolm Jayson MD FRCP
Qualified in Bristol in 1961. After a Rheumatology Consultancy there and at the RNHRD at Bath, he became Professor of Rheumatology in Manchester.

Jonas Kellgren MSc FRCP FRCS
Qualified at University College Hospital, London in 1934. After research work on 'pain' with Sir Thomas Lewis he served as a surgeon during the war. He was then appointed to the first Professorship in Rheumatology at Manchester. He was both a President and Orator of the Heberden Society and made major contributions to the study of pain and later generalised osteoarthritis.

Edward Calvin Kendall MS PhD DSc
He took his BSc in chemistry at Columbia University in 1908. He then worked as Director of the Department of Biochemistry at the Mayo Clinic where he synthesised glutathione. He proceeded to important work on thyroxine before launching into the steroid problems. In collaboration with Hench, Slocumb and Polley they isolated and proved the value of Compound E for which he obtained a Nobel Prize. He gave a Heberden Oration on Cortisone.

George Kersley OBE TD DL DSc MD FRCP
Qualified Cambridge and St Bartholomew's in 1931. He left St Bartholomew's to take up rheumatology at the Royal National Hospital for Rheumatic Diseases at Bath and later at the Bristol hospitals. He was on the original rheumatology committee of the College, a Founder Member of the ERC, of the Heberden Society when it became national, and of the BAPM. He was Adviser in Physical Medicine to the MEF during World War II and a President of the Heberden Society, the European League, and of the Physical Medical Section of the RSM. He was Mayor of Bath and Deputy Lieutenant of Avon and Vice President of the Conservative Medical Society.

Basil Kiernander MRCP D MRE
Qualified at Oxford and St Thomas's in 1936. He returned to the Radcliffe Hospital and was in charge of the Department of Physical Medicine. During World War II he was involved in rehabilitation work in the RAF.

Paul Klemperer
Born in 1887. He was originally a disciple of Freud and a member of the Psycho Analytic Society. This interest, however, eventually became a hobby, when he qualified as a Physician. He subsequently worked in the Wieden Spital in Vienna and in 1921 emigrated to America. He was appointed Associate Professor of Pathology in the Loyola Hospital in Chicago and subsequently moved to New York, where he became Professor of Pathology in the New York Postgraduate School of Medicine, and in 1926 moved to the Mount Sinai Hospital, where he remained for the rest of his active career. He was mainly responsible for the concept that connective tissues and their constituent collagen, play a very significant metabolic role in the pathology of rheumatic disease.

Richard Kovacs MD
Born 1884 was Professor of Physical Medicine at New York Polytechnic, wrote a standard text book on the subject and edited the *Year Books of Physical Medicine*. He was American Delegate to the International Congress held in London in 1936.

Hans Kraus MD
Of New York College of Medicine, he was particularly responsible for rehabilitation of back problems.

Frank Krusen MD
Born 1898, did research in physical medicine at the Mayo Clinic and wrote a standard text book on the subject in 1941. He was the first Chairman of the American Board of Physical Medicine and started the American Rehabilitation Foundation.

William Alexander Law OBE TD MD FRCS
Qualified at Cambridge and at the London Hospital in 1936. He was orthopaedic consultant to Oswestry, Hunterian Professor to the Royal College of Surgeons, a Watson Jones Lecturer and a Fellow of the British Orthopaedic Association. He was one of the first to satisfactorily carry out joint replacements with both hips at the same time and to accomplish osteotomy of the spine to correct gross curvature in ankylosing spondylitis.

John Lawrence MD FRCP
Qualified at Edinburgh 1930. At Manchester his interest turned to epidemiology, firstly with the Miner's Rheumatism Survey—he then

became Director of the ARC Field Unit. His Heberden Oration was on Rheumatoid Arthritis: Nature or Nurture—the Interplay of Genes in Sero-positive and Sero-negative Arthritis.

Frantisek Lenoch MD
Graduated at Prague University in 1923 and became Director of their Institute of Physical Medicine. Despite problems which arose because he would not join the Communist Party, he continued to hold his position and became President of the European League and was elected an Honorary Member of the Heberden Society.

Sydney Light MD
Worked at the Mount Sinai Hospital, New York and also at Boston and Yale. He compiled the *World Directory of Physical Medicine Specialists* in 1960.

Daniel McCarty MD FACP
Qualified in Pennsylvania 1954. In 1967 he became Professor of Medicine and Head of the Section of Arthritis and Metabolic Diseases in Chicago. He became President of the American Rheumatism Association. He did important work on calcium pyrophosphate dehydrate and gave his Oration on Crystals, Joints and Consternation.

Currier McEwen MD
Qualified in 1926 in New York where he became Professor. He was President of the American Rheumatism Association and did important early work on rheumatic fever.

David Linsay McKellan PhD FRCP
Qualified Cambridge and St Thomas's Hospital in 1966. After being a consultant in neurology, he was appointed Professor in Rehabilitation at Southampton.

Peter Maddison MD FRCP
Qualified Cambridge and St Bartholomew's in 1971 he became Consultant in Rheumatology at the Royal National Hospital for Rheumatic Diseases at Bath and in 1988 became Professor of Rheumatology for Bone and Joint Research, jointly at Bath University and the hospital.

RN Maini MD FRCP
Qualified Cambridge and Guy's in 1962. He became Professor of Immunological Rheumatology at Charing Cross Hospital and Director of Clinical Immunology at the Kennedy Institute. He was a Heberden Orator and a President of BLAR.

Michael Mason DM FRCP FRCS (Hon)
Qualified in Oxford and St Bartholomew's in 1942. He started his career in physical medicine at Chase Farm and then the London Hospital. He became Chairman of the ARC and was a President of the Heberden Society, of BARR and of BLAR. He died during the League Congress in San Francisco in 1977. The BSR has instituted a Michael Mason Medal in his memory.

JB Mennell MD
Qualified Cambridge and St Thomas's Hospital 1908 where he became Consultant Physiotherapist. He was probably the first modern physician to tackle manipulation of joints according to scientific principles.

John Moll DM PhD FRCP
Qualified and took his PhD and DM at Oxford and Leeds, before becoming a Consultant in Rheumatology at Sheffield. He is the author of the authorised *History of the Heberden Society*.

Charles Moran, The Rt Hon Sir Charles Lord Moran Kt MC MD PRCP
Qualified at St Mary's in 1908. He did much to put this hospital 'on the map' while Dean of the Medical School, when his success at fund raising earned him the name of 'Corkscrew Charlie'. He was well known as Personal Physician to Winston Churchill. His previous publication of his most valuable biography of Churchill caused some criticism. He was President of the Royal College of Physicians and was a Founder Honorary Member of the Heberden Society. His forte was more administration than research.

Helen Muir CBE DPhil DSc FRS FRCP (Hon)
She obtained her DPhil at Oxford in 1947 and then became Director of the Kennedy Institute where she was especially concerned with the study of the biochemistry of connective tissue and lysomal enzymes. She was an Orator and President of the Heberden Society.

Selwyn Nelson FRCP FRCPE FRACP FRCM
Qualified at Sydney in 1923. He was a President of the Australian Rheumatism and of the Physical Medicine and Rehabilitation Associations. He was the first President of SEAPAL in 1963 and was elected an Honorary Member of the Heberden Society.

Albert Neuberger CBE MD PhD FRS LLD PhD FRCP FRCP (Path)
He took his MD at Wurzburg and then came to Cambridge as a Beit Fellow in biochemistry. He became Head of the Biochemistry Department at the National Institute for Medical Research and Principal of the Wright Fleming Institute and the Lister Institute at Charing Cross. His Oration was on The Proteins of Connective Tissue and their Metabolism.

Desmond Newton MD FRCP
Qualified at St Thomas's Hospital in 1950 where he was involved in rehabilitation. He was a President of BARR.

George Nuki MD FRCP
Qualified 1966 at King's College Hospital, went to Cardiff as Reader and Consultant in Rheumatology and was then elected as Professor at Edinburgh University and Consultant to the Northern General Hospital. He was a Heberden Roundsman.

Charles O'Malley CVE MD
Born in Melbourne became Group Captain in the RAF where he was Director of Rehabilitation and started the unit at Torquay and then Loughborough and finally Garston Manor. He was Advisor to the Ministry of Health and World Veteran Association on Rehabilitation.

Henry Osmond-Clarke, Sir Henry KCVO CBE MCh FRCS
Qualified at the London Hospital. Became Air Commodore and was Hunterian Professor in 1956 and President of the British Orthopaedic Association in 1964 and was Consulting Orthopaedic Surgeon to HM The Queen.

Kit Wynn Parry MBE DM FRCP FRCS DPhys Med
Qualified at Oxford in 1947 and became a FRCS as well as FRCP. He was Director of Rehabilitation and Rheumatism at the Royal National Orthopaedic Hospital and was a Group Captain in the RAF, where he advised on rehabilitation.

James Waters Thornton 'Pat' Patterson MD FRCP
Was a Physician at Droitwich Spa, at the Arthur Stanley Institute of Rheumatic Diseases and member of the Research Body for the Correlation of Medical Science and Physical Education. He was ex-President of the section of Physical Medicine at the Royal Society of Medicine. Lieutenant Colonel of the Royal Army Medical Corps. Wrote papers on fibrositis and public health problems due to rheumatic diseases. Contributed to the *British Encyclopaedia of Medical Practice*.

Gabriel Panayi MD MRCP
Qualified Cambridge and Guy's Hospital in 1966. He won the Lionel Whitby Medal and then became Professor of Rheumatology at Guy's and then at London University.

Ralph Pemberton MD
Born 1877. Was the first American physician to call himself a rheumatologist and founded the rheumatology clinic at the Presbyterian Hospital Pennsylvania in 1926. He was Chairman of

the first American Committee for the Control of Rheumatism in 1927. He was President of La Ligue Contre le Rhumatism during World War II. A further note about his contribution to rheumatology will be found in the text.

Abou David Pollack MD
Pathologist who worked originally at the Mount Sinai Hospital in New York but subsequently had positions at various hospitals in Baltimore, culminating at the Johns Hopkins Hospital, working in collaboration with Drs Baehr and Klemperer. They published original work on the pathology of disseminated lupus erythematosus and other collagen diseases.

Arthur Porritt, The Lord Porritt GCMG PRCS FRCP
Born in New Zealand he qualified Oxford and St Mary's London in 1930. He was President of ARC for 17 years and President of the British Medical Association and Consultant Surgeon to the 21st Army Group. He then became Governor General of New Zealand and Surgeon to HM The Queen and King George VI.

Charles Ragan MD MACP
He took his MD at Columbia University in 1936 and became Professor of Medicine at the Presbyterian Hospital. He was a President of the American Rheumatism Association and was awarded a gold medal, largely for his work with Rose on the rheumatoid factor. He gave his Heberden Oration on Hypersensitivity in Rheumatoid Arthritis.

Matthew Ray DSO OBE MD MRCP
Qualified Edinburgh 1893. He was promoted Colonel and obtained a DSO in World War I. He worked as a spa physician at Harrogate and then came to Peto Place as senior physician. He was a Founder Member and later President of the Heberden Society and was awarded the OBE.

Arthur Richardson MD FRCP DPhys Med
Qualified in 1946. He worked in Physical Medicine at St Thomas's and Great Ormond Street Hospitals before becoming Director of the Department of Physical Medicine at the Royal Free. He was President of the BAPM (BARR).

Alessandro Robecchi MD
From Milan and Rome, he was one of the leading Italian rheumatologists of the 1960s and was President of both EULAR and ILAR.

Ray Robinson OBE FRACP
Qualified 1942 in Sydney and took a great interest in international

rheumatology including rheumatology in the third world countries. He was President both of ILAR and SEAPAL and an Honorary Member of the Heberden Society.

Johannes van Rood MD
Trained at Leiden and then Columbia University New York, qualifying 1952. He returned to become a Professor at Leiden and became a world authority on tissue typing and the HLA system. He gave his Oration on HLA as Regulator.

Howard Rusk MD
Was Director of Rehabilitation, New York Medical School. He was author of a text book on rehabilitation in 1958 and of *Living with Disability* and also papers on cardiovascular rehabilitation.

Oswald Savage OBE FRCP
Qualified at St Bartholomew's in 1932. For his war services as a Lieutenant Colonel he received his OBE. He then joined the Arthur Stanley Institute, the West London and the Kennedy Institute. He was a President of the Heberden Society.

The use of ACTH and the steroids and their dangers was one of his great interests.

Tom Scott MD FRCP
Qualified St Mary's Hospital 1949 and then worked at Hammersmith and Taplow. He became Consultant in Rheumatology at Charing Cross Hospital and the Kennedy Institute. A main interest of his was gout. He has been a President of the Heberden Society.

Jarvis Seegmiller MD
Starting his career in Chicago, he qualified in 1942. His interest was in biochemistry at Bethesda and he then became Director of Rheumatology at the University of California. His chief interest was then enzymology, which led him into the field of purine metabolism and gout on which he gave his Oration.

Hans Selye MD PhD DSc FRSC
Was born in 1907 in Vienna but spent most of his life in Montreal where he became Professor of Experimental Medicine. His greatest contribution was on the effect of stress on the endocrine system and on anaphylaxis, thus linking with the work in the 1940s of Hench and Kendall on adrenal and pituitary function. These two discoveries resulted in the development of the concept of the collagen diseases and brought rheumatology back into the mainstream of internal medicine. He gave a Heberden Oration on Stress and the General Adaptation Syndrome.

Stefan Sitaj MD DSc
Qualified at Bratislava and then became Director of the Research Institute at Piestany. Here he became a world authority on metabolic arthropathies and gave his Oration on Chondrocalcinosis and Ocronotic Arthropathy in 1973.

Morton Smart, Sir Morton KCVO DSO MD FRCP
Qualified at Edinburgh in 1902 and served in the South African War and World War I. He established the Electrical Department at Great Ormond Street Hospital and built up for himself a great private reputation especially for heliotherapy. He became the first Chairman on the formation of the BAPM.

Robert Stanton-Woods, Sir Robert KBE MD FRCP
Qualified at University College Hospital in 1904 and then moved to the London Hospital, where he established the first Department of Physical Medicine. He became a Founder Member of the BAPM.

Robert Stecker MD FACP
Took his MD at Harvard in 1923 and became Chief of the Arthritis Clinic at the Cleveland Metropolitan General Hospital. He became President of the American Rheumatism Association. He gave his Heberden Oration on Heberden's Nodes on which he did much genetic research.

George Storey MD FRCP
Qualified at the London Hospital in 1942 where he is in charge of the Physical Medicine Department, and is the authorised recorder of the History of Physical Medicine currently under production.

Roger Sturrock MD FRCP
Qualified in 1969 at the Westminster Hospital. After a lectureship in Nigeria, he became Professor in Rheumatic Diseases at Glasgow.

Nana Svartz
Qualified in Stockholm in 1918 and took her MD in 1927. Her early interest was in intestinal disease and in 1937 became Professor of Medicine at the Karolinska Institute. She then founded the Research Institute for Crippling Diseases, her special study being into rheumatoid arthritis. She sat on many international committees, including that for the Nobel Prize, and organised valuable conferences on rheumatic disease.

AK Thould MD FRCP
Qualified at St Bartholomew's in 1954. He is Editor of the *Annals of Rheumatic Diseases* and is President of the West Country Rheumatology Club. He was the 'founder' from Truro of Rheumatology in the South West of England.

Ronald Tunbridge, Sir Ronald OBE KBE MD FRCP
Qualified at Leeds in 1946. For his service in Malta as Adviser in Medicine he was awarded the OBE. He then became Professor of Medicine at Leeds. Among his many appointments was Vice-President of the Health Services Council for which he received the KBE. He was a President and Orator of the Heberden Society, President of the British Spas Federation and of the BMA. Apart from rheumatology, he contributed greatly to rehabilitation as author of the *Tunbridge Report* and had a special interest in cancer.

Kenneth Walton MD PhD DSc FRCP (Path)
Qualified at University College Hospital in 1942. He took up a career in pathology and became Professor of Pathology at Birmingham. He was a President of the Heberden Society. Apart from rheumatology, he did valuable work on lipid metabolism, arthrosclerosis and blood coagulation.

Reginald Watson-Jones, Sir Reginald MB FRCP MChir Orth
Orthopaedic surgeon to HM The Queen. Civilian Consultant in Orthopaedics to the RAF. Senior Vice-President of the Royal College of Surgeons. Hunterian Professor of the Royal College of Surgeons. Author of *Fractures and Joint Injuries*.

Lionel Whitby, Sir Lionel KCVO MC TD MD FRCP DPh
Qualified Cambridge and Middlesex Hospital in 1921 having already received his MC when he lost his leg at Paschendale. He became head of the Blood Transfusion Service during World War II. His great interest however was in bacteriology. He was Regius Professor of Physics and Vice-Chancellor of Cambridge University. He gave the first Heberden Round in 1948.

Derek Willoughby PhD DSc FRCP (Path)
Came from Cambridge to St Bartholomew's Hospital, where he became Professor of Experimental Pathology and later a Fellow of the Institute of Biologists and of the Royal College of Pathologists. His special interest was the pharmacology and cellular kinetics of inflammation and his Oration was on the Application of Animal Models.

Douglas Woolf MD FRCP DPhys Med
Qualified at the London Hospital in 1945 and took his DPhys Med in 1950. He joined the staff of the British Red Cross Society Clinic at Peto Place and then the Department of Rheumatology and Physical Medicine at the Middlesex. He played a very active role in the British Rheumatic Association and was their Chairman when they became Arthritis Care. He was also the part-time Medical Director of the Horder Homes.

Verna Wright MD FRCP
Qualified at Liverpool in 1953. He became Professor with a personal Chair in Rheumatology at Leeds. He was a President of the Heberden Society, BARR and Society for Back Pain Research. He was Adviser in Rheumatology to the DHSS. He took a special interest in engineering principles in joint movement. He did a great deal for Christian Youth.

DA Yates MD FRCP DPhys Med
Qualified at St Thomas's Hospital in 1953, where he became Director of the Department of Rheumatology. He was Consultant in Rheumatology to the Army and was the last President of BARR before it was amalgamated with the Heberden Society to form the BSR.

Morris Ziff PhD MD FACP
Qualified in New York in 1937. His early leanings were towards chemistry and biochemistry but he later became Professor of Rheumatology at Texas University. He was President of the American Rheumatism Association and gave his Heberden Oration on Immunologic Aspects of Connective Tissue Disorders.

Appendices

MEETINGS AND PRESIDENTS OF THE LEAGUES

La Ligue Contre Le Rhumatism

1925	International Rheumatism Committee of ISMH	Dr Fortescue Fox
1928	Ligue formed at Buxton	
1929	First Congress, Budapest	Professor Baron Koran
1930	Liege	Professor Gunzburg
1932	Paris	Professor Benzancon
1934	Moscow	Professor Konchalovsky
1936	Lund and Stockholm	Professor Ingvar
1938	Oxford and Bath	Sir Faquahar Buzzard
		Lord Horder
1947	Copenhagen	Dr Weil

The International League (ILAR)

1949	New York	Dr Ralph Pemberton & Dr R Freyberg
1953	Geneva	Professor Jarlov & Dr R Stecher
1957	Toronto	Professor Florent Coste & Dr W Graham
1961	Rome	Professor Robles-Gil
1965	Mar del Plata	Professor Alessandro Robecchi
1969	Prague	Professor Harrera-Ramos
1973	Kyoto	Dr Pedro Barcelo
1977	San Francisco	Dr Ray Robinson
1981	Paris	Dr EP Engleman
1985	Sydney	Professor J Villiaumey
1989	Rio de Janeiro	Kenneth Muirden

European League (EULAR)

1947	Copenhagen	Professor Edstrom
1951	Barcelona	Professor Weil
		Dr Copeman
1955	Schevenigen	Dr Ferond
		Dr Pedro Barcelo
1959	Istanbul	Professor Johan Hans Goslings
		Dr Forestier
1963	Stockholm	Professor Alessandro Robecchi
		Professor Edstrom

1967 Lisbon	Professor Lenoch
	Dr Kersley
1971 Brighton	Professor Gotsch
	Professor de Seze
1975 Helsinki	Professor Laine
	Professor Tzonchev
1979 Weisbaden	Professor Boni
	Professor Bywaters
1983 Moscow	Professor Nassonova
1987 Athens	Professor Mathies
	Professor Pipitone
1991 Budapest	Professor Lequesue
	Dr Barnes

The Pan American League (PANLAR)

1944	R Pemberton
1949	Ruiz Moreno
1955 Rio de Janeiro	R Freyberg
1959 Washington	W Graham
1963 Santiago de Chile	P Nava
1967 Mexico City	F Valenzuela Ravest
1971 Caracas	P Martinez Elezondo
1974 Toronto	O Garcia Morteo
1978 Bogota	
1982 Washington	
1986 Buenos Aires	
1990 Guadalajara	

South East Asian, Pacific & Australasian League (SEAPAL)

1963	Selwyn Nelson
1968	Ray Robinson
1972 Auckland	M Desai
1976 Singapore	S Sasaki
1980 Manila	
1984 Bangkok	
1988 Tokyo	
1992 Bali	

British League Against Rheumatism (BLAR)

1977	Dr Michael Mason
1981	Dr CG Barnes
1985	Professor RN Maini
1989	Dr Rodney Grahame

BRITISH ASSOCIATION OF PHYSICAL MEDICINE, (BAPM) LATER THE BRITISH ASSOCIATION FOR RHEUMATOLOGY AND REHABILITATION (BARR)

Past Presidents

1943-45 The Lord Horder
1956-59 Philippe Bauwens
1959-62 Hugh Burt
1962-65 William Tegner
1965-68 Frank Cooksey
1968-71 Michael Mason
1971-74 Archibald Boyle
1974-76 Desmond Newton
1976-78 Tony Richardson
1978-80 Verna Wright
1980-84 DA Yates

BRITISH SOCIETY OF RHEUMATOLOGY (BSR)

1984-86 George Nuki
1986-88 Rodney Grahame
1989-91 Ian Haslock
1991   RN Maini
          Michael Snaith

PRESIDENTS, ORATORS AND ROUNDSMEN OF THE HEBERDEN SOCIETY

Presidents of the Heberden Society

1936	Dr Frank D Howitt
1937	Dr Matthew B Ray
1938	Dr CB Heald
1939-46	Dr Charles W Buckley
1947	Mr Sydney L Higgs
1948	Mr Sydney L Higgs
1949	Dr Will SC Copeman
1950	Dr Will SC Copeman
1951	The Rt Hon The Lord Cohen of Birkenhead
1952	The Rt Hon The Lord Cohen of Birkenhead
1953	The Rt Hon The Lord Horder
1954	Professor Sir Ronald E Tunbridge
1955	Professor Sir Ronald E Tunbridge
1956	Dr Ernest Fletcher
1957	Dr Ernest Fletcher
1958	Professor Jonas H Kellgren
1959	Professor Jonas H Kellgren
1960	Dr F Dudley Hart
1961	Dr F Dudley Hart
1962	Dr George D Kersley
1963	Dr George D Kersley
1964	Professor Eric GL Bywaters
1965	Professor Eric GL Bywaters
1966	Dr Oswald Savage
1967	Dr Oswald Savage
1968	Professor Ian JR Duthie
1969	Professor Ian JR Duthie
1970	Dr Alan GS Hill
1971	Dr Alan GS Hill
1972	Dr Leonard E Glynn
1973	Dr Allan St J Dixon
1974	Dr R Michael Mason
1975	Dr Barbara Ansell
1976	Professor Kenneth W Walton
1977	Professor Verna Wright
1978	Professor John Ball
1979	Dr J Tom Scott
1980	Professor Helen Muir
1981	Professor Harry J Currey
1982	Dr Clifford F Hawkins
1983	Dr Derrick Brewerton

Heberden Orators (Medallists)

1938	Dr Ernest Fletcher
1939	Dr William SC Copeman
1942	Dr Philip S Hench
1949	Professor F Wood Jones
1950	Professor Hans Selye
1951	Professor Edward C Kendall
1952	The Rt Hon The Lord Horder
1953	Sir W Russell Brain
1954	Dr Robert M Stecker
1955	Professor Walter Bauer
1956	Professor Sir Ronald Tunbridge
1957	Professor Knud Brochner-Mortensen
1958	Dr Charles Ragan
1959	Professor Albert Neuberger
1960	Dr Joseph J Bunim
1961	The Rt Hon The Lord Cohen of Birkenhead
1962	Dr Jacques Forestier
1963	Professor Jonas H Kellgren
1964	Dr Morris Ziff
1965	Sir Austin Bradford Hill
1966	Professor Eric GL Bywaters
1967	Dr Leonard E Glynn
1968	Dame Honor Fell
1969	Dr John S Lawrence
1970	Professor John Ball
1971	Professor Dugald L Gardner
1972	Dr Anthony C Allison
1973	Professor Stefan Sitaj
1974	Professor Derek A Willoughby
1975	Dr Lawrence E Shulman
1976	Dr Helen Muir
1977	Dr Barbara M Ansell
1978	Dr John T Dingle
1979	Professor Jarvis E Seegmiller
1980	Professor Stephen M Crane
1981	Dr Roy M Acheson
1982	Professor Daniel J McCarty
1983	Professor Johannes J Van Rood
1984	Dr L Thomas
1985	Professor Verna Wright
1986	Dr P Latchman
1987	Dr F Austin
1988	Professor R Maini
1989	Professor Hans Valkenberg
1990	Professor N Zvaifler

Heberden Roundsmen
(With which is associated a Medal, presented by Dr AGS Hill in 1972)

1948	Sir Lionel Whitby	Addenbrookes Hospital, Cambridge
1949	Professor LJ Whitts	The Radcliffe Infirmary, Oxford
1950	Professor F Coste	Hôpital Cochin, Paris
1951	Professor Sir Stanley Davidson	Royal Infirmary, Edinburgh
1952	Professor Sir Henry Cohen	Royal Infirmary, Liverpool
1953	Professor JH Kellgren	University of Manchester
1954	Professor SJ Hartfall	General Infirmary, Leeds
1955	Dr F Dudley Hart	Westminster Medical School, London
1956	Dr GD Kersley	Royal United Hospital, Bath
1957	Professor IJR Duthie	Northern General Hospital, Edinburgh
1958	Professor J Gosling	University Hospital, Leiden, Holland
1959	Professor EGL Bywaters	Royal Postgraduate Medical School, London
1960	Dr WS Tegner	The London Hospital
1961	Dr Oswald Savage	West London Hospital
1962	Dr AGS Hill	Stoke Mandeville Hospital
1963	Dr HF West	Sheffield University
1964	Professor GA Smart & Dr Malcolm Thompson	The Royal Victoria Infirmary, Newcastle-upon-Tyne
1965	Dr James Sharp	Devonshire Royal Hospital, Buxton
1966	Dr RM Mason	The London Hospital
1967	Dr Barbara Ansell	Canadian Red Cross Hospital, Taplow
1968	Dr CF Hawkins	Queen Elizabeth Hospital, Birmingham
1969	Dr A St J Dixon	Royal National Hospital for Rheumatic Diseases, Bath
1970	Dr WRM Alexander	Northern General Hospital, Edinburgh
1971	Dr JT Scott	The Kennedy Institute, London
1972	Professor HLF Currey	The London Hospital
1973	Professor V Wright	Rheumatism Research Unit, Leeds
1974	Dr EBD Hamilton	King's College Hospital, London
1975	Dr N Cardoe	Norfolk and Norwich Hospital, Norwich
1976	Professor W Watson Buchanan	The Centre for Rheumatic Diseases, Glasgow

1977 Dr KN Lloyd   Welsh National School of
                             Medicine, Cardiff
1978 Dr Logie Bain   The Medical School, Aberdeen
1979 Dr John Cosh   Royal National Hospital, Bath
1980 Dr HW Balme   St Bartholomew's Hospital,
                             London
1981 Dr AM Denman   Northwick Park, London
1982 Dr GR Hughes   Royal Postgraduate Medical
                             School, London
1983 Professor G Nuki   Northern General Hospital,
                             Edinburgh
1984 Professor P Dieppe   Bristol Royal Infirmary
1985 Professor P Bacon   Queen Elizabeth Hospital,
                             Birmingham
1986 Dr L Holt   Royal Infirmary, Manchester
1987 Dr B Bresnigham   University College, Dublin
1988 Dr Huskisson   St Bartholomew's Hospital,
                             London
1989 Dr Michael Snaith   Middlesex Hospital, London
1990 Dr Ian Griffiths   Royal Victoria Infirmary,
                             Newcastle on Tyne
1991 Dr AG Mowat   Nuffield Orthopaedic Centre,
                             Oxford

SOME IMPORTANT DATES IN THE HISTORY OF BRITISH RHEUMATOLOGY AND REHABILITATION

1742	Opening of The Bath Hospital, becoming the Royal Mineral Water Hospital and then the Royal National Hospital for Rheumatic Diseases, Bath
1826	The Royal Bath Hospital, Harrogate
1858	The Royal Devonshire Hospital, Buxton
1917	First Physical Medicine Department at the London Hospital
1921	The International Society of Medical Hydrology [published *Archives of Med Hydrol* (1922-39)]
1925	Foundation of ISMH Rheumatology Committee
1928	ISMH Rheumatology Committee became La Ligue Contre le Rhumatism [published *Acta Rheumatologica* (1929-39)]
1924-28	Dr Alison Glover's *Reports*
1930	The Peto Place BRCS Clinic for Hydrology and Rheumatology
1931	The Physical Medicine Section of the Royal Society of Medicine formed from the Balneological and Climatological Section (1907)
1934	Royal College of Physicians Rheumatology Committee [published *Reports* (1934-36)]
1936	Empire Rheumatism Council ERC (published *Reports*, which became the *Annals* in 1944)
1937	Heberden Society formed from the staff committee of the Peto Place Clinic
1937	Opening of the Rheumatology units at St John's and St Elizabeth's and St Stephen's Hospitals, London
1938	Rheumatology Unit at The West London Hospital
1943	The British Association of Physical Medicine BAPM
1947	Taplow Hospital
1947	The British Rheumatic Association BRA
1948	The Arthur Stanley Institute formed from the Peto Red Cross Clinic
1948	Diploma in Physical Medicine awarded by the Royal College of Physicians
1948	The Rheumatism Research Unit for the SW and Oxford Regions at Bath
1952	First ERC Fellow appointed at Sheffield
1953	First Chair in Rheumatology at Manchester, Professor Kellgren
1954	Field Unit in Epidemiology of Rheumatic Disease, Manchester
1957	Chair in Rheumatology, Post Graduate Hospital, London, Professor Bywaters

1959	Chair in Rheumatology, Edinburgh, Professor Duthie
1959	Industrial Unit for Rheumatology, Edinburgh
1959	Electron Microscopy Unit, St Thomas's Hospital, London
1963	The British Association of Manipulative Medicine
1964	The Empire Rheumatism Council, having budded off the Canadian, Australian and New Zealand Councils became the Arthritis and Rheumatism Council (ARC)
1965	The Arthur Stanley Institute became the Department of Rheumatology-Rehabilitation at the Middlesex Hospital; Chair in Rheumatology at the Kennedy Institute, London
1969	The Back Pain Association
1970	The BAPM became the British Association for Rheumatology and Rehabilitation BARR
1971	The Back Pain Society
1971	Chair in Rheumatology, Leeds, Professor V Wright
1972	Chair in Rheumatology, Glasgow, Professor Buchanan
1972	The Bone and Joint Unit, the London Hospital
1974	The Physical Medicine Section of the RSM became the Section of Rheumatology and Rehabilitation
1974	Chair in Rheumatology, the London Hospital, Professor Currey; Chair in Rehabilitation, Southampton, Professor Ville; Chair in Rehabilitation, Leeds, Professor Aitken
1977	World Rheumatism Year
1979	Chair in Rheumatology, Manchester, Professor Malcolm Jayson
1981	Chair in Rheumatology, Birmingham, Professor Paul Bacon
1983	Fusion of the Heberden Society and BARR to become the British Society for Rheumatology BSR
1987	Chair in Rheumatology, Bristol, Professor P Dieppe
1988	Chair in Rheumatology at RNHRD, Bath, Professor P Maddison; Chair in Rehabilitation at Leeds, Professor Chamberlain
1990	Chair in Rheumatology at Leeds, Professor Sturrock
1991	Chair in Rheumatology at Guy's Hospital, London, Professor Penayi

NOTES ON THE HISTORY OF UNITS IN THE UK WITH PROFESSORIAL CHAIRS IN RHEUMATOLOGY AND REHABILITATION

Rheumatology

Bath, Professor Peter Maddison
Rheumatology in Bath dates back to the change in name of the Mineral Water Hospital founded in 1742, to that of the Royal National Hospital for Rheumatic Diseases in 1936. In 1948 the Research Unit of the South West and Oxford Region was formed with George Kersley as Director, the Oxford element later being split off under the directorship of Alan Hill. Under the chairmanship of Alan Dixon, the Bath Institute for Rheumatic Diseases was opened by Lord Hailsham in 1984. In 1989 the hospital was granted a Royal coat of arms incorporating a tripod indicating treatment, teaching and research. A department to cover these three aspects of rehabilitation was given national status in 1974 with Tony Clarke as Director. In 1988 Peter Maddison was established as the Glaxo Professor of Osteoarticular Pathology, jointly with Bath University and the Royal National Hospital.

Birmingham, Professor Paul Bacon
The Department of Rheumatology in Birmingham was set up in 1981, within the Department of Medicine, with the appointment of Paul Bacon to the new ARC Chair in Rheumatology. It incorporated the laboratory facilities of the Department of Investigative Pathology, directed by Kenneth Walton who retired the following year. The ARC endowment was backed by the NHS, who had recognised the West Midlands as a rheumatologically deprived Region. Since then, the Department has expanded and become a full university department with a strong research bias. The first Senior Lecturer was David Blake, who went on to the Chair at the London Hospital. New appointments have included Paul Emery, Senior Lecturer in Adult Rheumatology; Taunton Southwood, as the first Senior Lecturer in Paediatric Rheumatology in the UK; Hill Gaston as Senior Research Fellow/Consultant; and Stephen Young as New Blood Non-Clinical Lecturer.

The Department has laboratory space in the Clinical Research Block of the Medical School. Research centres on the involvement of T cells in the pathogenesis of chronic inflammatory rheumatic disease and in the systemic connective tissue diseases. Laboratory research involves cell biology with increasing emphasis on molecular biology and the use of MR spectroscopy to examine protein/protein interactions.

Bristol, Professor Paul Dieppe
For many years, Bristol relied on Bath for some cover in rheumatology with George Kersley doing sessions at the Bristol Royal

and Southmead Hospitals and as lecturer in Physical Medicine to the University. Dr Malcolm Jason was appointed jointly to the staff of the Bath Royal National Hospital and as Lecturer to the Professor of Medicine at Bristol. He was succeeded by Paul Dieppe who in 1987 relinquished his Bath appointment and became Professor of Rheumatology at Bristol University with ARC support. With John Kirwan as Senior Lecturer, Bristol has been especially interested in degenerative joint disease and crystal arthropathies.

Edinburgh, Professor George Nuki
The Edinburgh Rheumatic Diseases Unit was opened in 1947 at the Northern General Hospital under the direction of Dr IJR Duthie as Consultant Rheumatologist and Honorary Senior Lecturer in the University. In 1955 a new outpatient department and research laboratories were built with a capital grant from the Oliver Bird Fund of the Nuffield Foundation and in 1963 this accommodation was extended by the addition of the McFarlane Wing with funding from the ERC. Ian Duthie was promoted to Honorary Readership in 1964 and awarded a Personal Chair in the University of Edinburgh in 1968.

After Professor Duthie retired in 1977, the University established the ARC Chair in Rheumatology within the Department of Medicine of the Western General Hospital at the Northern General Hospital. Professor George Nuki was appointed as the first incumbent in 1979. The Rheumatic Diseases Unit laboratories at the Northern General Hospital were extended in 1981 to provide cell culture and biochemical research facilities with further funding from the ARC. Research at the Rheumatic Diseases Unit has included basic research into the pathogenesis of rheumatoid arthritis, osteoarthritis, gout and disorders of purine metabolism, and clinical studies on bone mass in rheumatic diseases. Dr Gordon Duff was promoted to Senior Lecturer in 1987 and directed an ARC supported molecular immunology group until he was appointed to the Lord Florey Chair of Molecular Medicine in the University of Sheffield in 1990. Professor Dugald Gardner, who had worked in Edinburgh during the early years of the Rheumatic Diseases Unit, returned to Edinburgh in 1989 to found an osteoarticular pathology laboratory.

Over the years the Rheumatic Diseases Unit has worked closely with the orthopaedic surgeons at the Princess Margaret Rose Hospital and the Arthritis Surgery Research Unit (directed by Mr WA Souter) has played a leading role in the development of arthritis surgery and prosthetic joints. The Rheumatic Diseases Unit has clinical, teaching and training links with the Rehabilitation Unit directed by Professor Cairns Aitken.

Glasgow, Professor Roger Sturrock
The Centre for Rheumatic Diseases in Glasgow was opened in 1975 with Dr Watson Buchanan, later Professor Buchanan, as its first

Clinical Director. Dr Tony Boyle was the first member of Professor Buchanan's staff and subsequently Dr Carson Dick joined the Unit as an NHS Consultant in Rheumatology. The Centre for Rheumatic Diseases consisted of 39 beds and soon began to act as a Regional Referral Centre for Rheumatic Disease patients in the West of Scotland. In 1984 it moved into the Royal Infirmary in Glasgow. In 1990, as a result of the McLeod Bequest, together with a grant from the ARC, the McLeod/ARC Chair of Rheumatology was established. Roger Sturrock was appointed to the Chair in December of 1990 and this appointment will enable more research facilities to be available for rheumatology.

Guy's Hospital, London, Professor Gabriel Panayi
At Guy's Hospital, the Department of Physical Medicine was founded by Dr E Crisp, succeeded by Dr P Hume Kendall and then Dr H Burry. Dr Rodney Grahame was appointed in 1969 and the name of the Department changed to that of Rheumatology. In 1973, Dr Gabriel Panayi became ARC Lecturer in Rheumatology and succeeded to the ARC Chair in 1979, which later covered Guy's and St Thomas's Hospitals. In 1990, Dr Grahame became Professor of Clinical Rheumatology to the University of London.

Rheumatology at Guy's has had a special interest in cellular immunology and immunogenetics and has special clinics for spondylitis, athletics, immunotherapy, gout, paediatrics, back pain and psoriatic arthritis.

Kennedy Institute, London, Professor Tiny Maini
The Kennedy Institute was founded in 1965 thanks to the benefaction of Mr and Mrs Kennedy and largely at the instigation of Will Copeman. Their first Director was DL Gardiner in 1966, who left to become Professor of Pathology in Belfast in 1972. He was followed by LE Glynn and then Helen Muir, who became Professor of Pathology at London University in 1990. Professor AN Maini has now taken over the reins as Director. Drs Oswald Savage and Tom Scott have been clinical physicians to the Institute.

The main divisions of the Institute are now Biochemistry, Clinical Immunology and Cellular Biology. The ARC has, from the beginning, been the main contributor to research grants and management.

Leeds, Professor Verna Wright
Rheumatology practice was first undertaken at Leeds by Dr SJ Hartfall, Professor of Clinical Medicine, with Dr Hugh Garland and Dr William Goldie. Hartfall was the first to use gold in England in the treatment of rheumatoid arthritis. Many years later a controlled trial by the ERC showed this treatment to be effective. His rheumatological in-patient beds were at the Regional Rheumatology Centre at Harrogate, which at that time had well over 200 beds.

This has gradually been reduced to 25% of that level. Dr V Wright was appointed as a Clinical Assistant to Professor Hartfall and on his retirement Dr Wright took over the rheumatological side of the Department.

A personal Chair was awarded by the University to Dr Wright in 1970, and this was endowed by the ARC in 1988. The Unit developed along a number of lines so that the Department has four divisions. One is a clinical sciences group looking particularly at aspects of seronegative polyarthritis, osteoarthritis and non-articular rheumatism. A bioengineering group (head, Dr BB Seedhom) has been established looking at the stiffness of joints, the properties of normal and diseased articular cartilage, the replacement of joints and ligaments, and the transmissibility of the spine to vibration. A clinical pharmacology unit (head, Dr HA Bird) is established at Leeds with laboratories at the Royal Bath Hospital in Harrogate. The fourth division is that of rehabilitation and is headed by Professor MA Chamberlain.

The Royal London Hospital, Professor David Blake
Rheumatology and Rehabilitation at the London Hospital goes back to 1917 with the formation of a Remedial Gymnastic, Electrotherapy and Massage Department under Robert Stanton Woods. In 1935 six beds were allocated and in 1955 William Tegner and Michael Mason succeeded Sir Robert. In 1965 the department was renamed the Department of Physical Medicine and Rheumatology with Harry Currey, shortly to have a personal Chair in 1970, as head of the ARC Bone and Joint Research Unit. This worked closely with the Department of Pathology and Orthopaedics. In 1976 the ARC funded a new building to house the Bone and Joint Unit. In 1968 Colin Barnes was appointed Consultant in Rheumatology and now heads the NHS team. In 1987, on the retirement of Professor Currey, Dr Blake succeeded him in the ARC Chair of Rheumatology and he now heads the academic Department of Rheumatology, which covers research into inflammatory mechanisms, heredity, experimental pathology, orthopaedics and clinical rheumatology.

Manchester, Professor Malcolm Jayson
The Manchester Rheumatology Centre was started in 1947 with the appointment of Professor Kellgren as Clinical Director. In 1953 an ARC Chair was instituted, the first in Rheumatology in the UK. At the same time, John Chapman was appointed to start the Electron Microscopy Unit and a year later John Lawrence became Director of the Epidemiology Unit at the behest of the miners and backed by the ARC. He was followed by Philip Wood and Alan Silman.

In 1978, John Ball received a Personal Chair in Osteoarticular Pathology to continue his work on the rheumatoid factor and enthesopathies in ankylosing spondylitis. David Jackson became

Professor of Medical Biochemistry, working closely with the rheumatology research. In 1977 Malcolm Jayson succeeded Professor Kellgren and the Department of Rheumatology has now moved to Salford. It covers the full range of 'rheumatic' disease, including back pain, pain perception, psychological factors and rehabilitation.

Rehabilitation

Edinburgh, Professor Cairns Aitken
Professor Cairns Aitken was appointed to the Chair of Rehabilitation Studies in 1974. The Chair had been endowed by the National Fund for Research into Crippling Diseases, the Thistle Foundation and the Hugh Fraser Foundation. The Rehabilitation Studies Unit was affiliated with the Department of Orthopaedic Surgery at the Princess Margaret Rose Hospital at Fairmilehead, Edinburgh. Services were also developed at the Astley Ainslie Hospital in Edinburgh. These were more concerned with cardiac and neurological disorders as well as locomotor disorders. Three additional consultants were appointed, one being a rheumatologist, Dr John Hunter, who had trained in Manchester.

The Rehabilitation Studies Unit has obtained nearly £2m in grants, the largest amount from the Association of British Insurers. This has funded work on compensation for personal injury, led by a social scientist, Dr Paul Cornes. Dr Cornes is Editor of the *International Journal of Rehabilitation Research*. Both he and Professor Aitken have been elected to serve as Presidents of the Society for Research in Rehabilitation. Professor Aitken is now the Dean of the Faculty of Medicine.

Leeds, Professor Marcella Chamberlain
The Chair of Rheumatological Rehabilitation at Leeds was endowed by the Charterhouse Clinic Foundation in 1988 with Marcella Anne Chamberlain as Professor. She had previously been in charge of the Juvenile Chronic Arthritis Clinic at Leeds. The chief interests of the Rehabilitation Unit are Rheumatology, Clinical Pharmacology, Bioengineering and Rehabilitation, concentrating on physically handicapped school leavers and the effectiveness of the services provided. Vera Newmann has been appointed as consultant to the department.

Southampton, Professor Linsay McKellan
Following on with the work in rheumatology by Michael Crawley, a combined rheumatology and physical medicine clinic was started in Southampton in 1950. In 1974 Professor Glanville started a Rehabilitation Unit. When the new General Hospital was opened, there were 14 beds for rheumatology (Dr Armstrong and Dr Ellis)

and 17 beds for rehabilitation, with Professor L McKellan, previously a neurologist, in charge. The particular interest of the unit is Community Care, Head Injuries and Parkinson's Disease.

From examination of these notes on the Professorial Units in Rheumatology and Rehabilitation, it should be noted that seven Chairs in Rheumatology have come into being in three years. Likewise, the three Chairs in Rehabilitation have been recruited from diverse sources, as was suggested for Rheumatology by the Royal College of Physicians many years ago—from pure rheumatology, general medicine, orthopaedics or physical medicine. In rehabilitation the Chairs have been filled by a rheumatologist (Leeds), a psychiatrist (Edinburgh) and a neurologist (Southampton). The latter appointment is in line with the number of neurological cases now being dealt with by many rehabilitation departments.

Index

Abrahams, Sir Adolf 7
acroparaesthesiae 78
Acta Rheumatologica (see La Ligue)
agranulocytosis 87
Allopurinol 84, 91
Alton Orthopaedic Hospital 4
American Association for the Control of Rheumatism (AACR) 71
  Rheumatism Reviews 71
American Association for the Study and Control of Rheumatic Diseases 71
American Board of Physical Medicine 76
American Committee for the Control of Rheumatism 71
American Congress of Physical Medicine and Rehabilitation 75
American Physiotherapy Association 74
American Rehabilitation Foundation Policy Group 76
American Rheumatism Association (ARA) 12, 14, 71-74
American Rheumatism Foundation 72-74
amidopyrin 86
amputation 22
Andrews, Michael 33
ankylosing spondylitis 22, 57, 87
ankylosing vertebral hyperstosis (Forestier's disease) 42
Annals of Physical Medicine (see BARR)
Annals of the Rheumatic Diseases 31, 35, 40, 102
Ansell, Barbara 65
Anturan 84
aplastic anaemia 87
Archives of Medical Hydrology (see ISMH)

arthritides 22
arthritis 77, 83
Arthritis Care 29, 68, 73
Arthritis and Rheumatism Council (ARC) 18, 31, 33, 35, 52, 68, 73
Arthur Stanley Institute (see Stanley, Arthur)
Aschoff, L 22
aspirin 58, 83
Association of Physicians of Great Britain and Ireland 35, 37
Association of Physical Medicine 102
azathioprin 90

Bach, Francis 29, 33, 48, 68
Back Pain Society 18, 69
Baehr, George 23, 56
Bailey, LB 49
Bain, Dr Logie 68
balneotherapy 1
Bannatyne, GA 1
Bath 1, 6, 25
  Bath Hospital 1, 3
  Bellotts Hospital 3
  Royal Mineral Water Hospital (Min) 1, 29, 43
  Royal National Hospital for Rheumatic Diseases 1, 6, 30, 43, 52, 53, 55, 64, 95
  Royal United Hospital 6, 29, 53, 55
  Wolfson Research Centre 53
Bath Hospital (see Bath)
Barbor, Dr 70
Barker 19
Barnes, Colin G 18, 33
Baruch 18, 50
Bauer, Dr Walter 41, 72
Bauwens, Dr Phillipe 49, 50, 63
Bellotts Hospital (see Bath)
Benemid 22, 84
Bevan, Aneuran 51, 58

Beveridge 51
blood dyscrasias 83
Bochenek, Miss Cecilia 69
Bouillaud 22
Bourgnignon 50
Bowen, AC 68
Boyle, Dr AC 18
Van Breemen, J 9, 10-12, 18
British Association of Manipulative Medicine (BAMM) 19, 69
British Association of Physical Medicine (BAPM) 18, 26, 48-50, 54, 55, 61, 62, 99
  Journal of Physical Medicine and Industrial Hygiene 50
  Journal of Rheumatology and Rehabilitation 50
British Association of Rheumatology and Rehabilitation (BARR) 50, 62, 102
  Annals of Physical Medicine 102
  British Journal of Rheumatology 102
  Rheumatology and Physical Medicine 102
  Rheumatology and Rehabilitation 102
British Balneological and Climatological Society 42
British Council for Rehabilitation of the Disabled 18
British Journal of Rheumatology
  (see BARR)
  (see BSR)
British League Against Rheumatism (BLAR) 17, 18, 65
British Medical Association (BMA) 37, 53
British Orthopaedic Association 23
British Orthopaedic Society 23
British Rheumatic Association 56, 68
British Rheumatism Association (BRA) 29, 33, 73
British Rheumatism and Arthritis Association (BRAA) 18, 68
British Society for Rheumatology (BSR) 42, 62, 102
  British Journal of Rheumatology 102

British Spas Federation 26
Brochner-Mortensen, Kund 42
Buckley, Charles B 31, 40, 43
Bunim, Joe 42
Burt, Barnes 30, 43
Burt, Hugh 39
Butazolidin 84, 87
Buxton 3
Buxton Bath Charity 3
Bywaters, Eric 35, 41, 54, 55, 65

Cairns, Sir Hugh 66
calcitonin 79
Canadian Red Cross Hospital, Taplow 65
Capener, Norman 30
carcinomatosis 22, 79
carpal tunnel compression syndrome 78
Di Caspero 18
Causation and Treatment of Chronic Rheumatism (see Fox, R Fortescue)
Charing Cross Hospital, London 65
Charnley, John 23
  vitallium head and polyethylene socket 24
Chartered Society of Physiotherapists 35
Charterhouse Clinic 42
Chaselycot, Eastbourne 67
Cheyne, George 1
chlorambucil 90
chloroquine (see Mepacrin)
cholera 4
chondrocalcinosis 22, 78
Churchill, The Rt Hon Winston 31
cinchophen 22, 84
Clarke, Dr Tony 95
Clemmesen 49, 50
Coates, Vincent 9, 30
Cohen, Sir Henry, later Lord Cohen of Birkenhead 7, 35, 37, 39, 40
colchicine 22, 83, 84
Committee for the Study and Control of Rheumatism 12
Committee for the Study and Investigation of Rheumatism 35
Committee for the Study of Rheumatology 9, 11
condylar knee prosthesis 24

Cooksey, Frank 45, 48-50, 54
Copeman, William 14, 17, 28, 29, 31, 33-37, 40, 54, 55, 65, 68
corticosteroids 56, 57, 72, 79, 80, 84, 85, 90
corticotrophin 84
cortisone 22, 54, 57, 60, 68, 85
Crowe, Dr Warren 42
Cumberbatch 18
Currey, Harry 65
cyclophosphamide 90
Cyriax, Dr James 62, 70

Dainton, Lord 33, 34
Davidson, Dr John 70
Davidson, Sir Stanley 39, 83
Devonshire, Duke of 3
Diagnosis Related Groups (DRG) 97
Dieppe 22
Dietrich 9
dimercaptopropanol 89
diphosphonates 79
Diploma in Medical Rehabilitation (see Royal College of Physicians)
Diploma of Physical Medicine (see Royal College of Physicians)
Diploma of Rehabilitation Medicine 102
discoid lupus erythematosus 88, 89
disseminated sclerosis 96
Dixon, Allan St John 14, 69
Dorset House Occupational Therapy Centre 50
Droitwich 4
Duchess of Gloucester Hospital, Isleworth 67
Duthie, IJ 39

Ebbetts, Dr John 70
Edgecombe 43
Edinburgh, Duke of 68
Edstrom, Professor 14
Elizabeth, HM The Queen 30
Emergency Medical Services (EMS) 33
Empire Rheumatism Council (ERC) 26, 29, 31, 33, 35, 60, 83

EMS Rehabilitation Service 54
Enham Village Centre 11
enteropathic arthritis 79
eosinophilic fasciitis 79
European League Against Rheumatism (EULAR) 14, 15, 18
exfoliative dermatitis 83

fibromyalgia 25, 79
'fibrositis' 25
Finsen 18
Fletcher, Ernest 41
Forestier, Henri 42, 83, 88
Forestier, Jacques 9, 10, 18, 42, 83, 88
Forestier's disease (see ankylosing vertebral hyperostosis)
Fraser, Professor Sir Francis 26, 31, 65
Fox, Dr R Fortescue 9, 10, 31, 39
Causation and Treatment of Chronic Rheumatism 11
Fox, Sir Theodor 10, 31, 33
Freeman, Michael 24
Freyberg, Richard 14, 76

Galen 1
Garrod 22
Garston Manor 50
Gauvain, Sir Henry 4
General Medical Council 37
George, King 39
Girdlestone excision 23
Gloucester, Duke of 31, 34
Glover, Alison 21, 31
Reports on the Incidence of the Rheumatic Diseases (1924-28) 21, 31, 40
Godber, Sir George 56
gold 21, 42, 83, 88, 89
gout 1, 22, 42, 57, 83, 87, 91
Gowers, Sir William 25
Grundy, Mr Stanley 69
Gunzburg 9, 10
Guttmann, Ludwig 66, 67

haematemesis 83
Hammersmith Postgraduate Hospital 65

Harewood, Lord 4
Hargraves 22
Harrogate 3, 8
Hart, 'Frank' Dudley 41
Heald, CB 34, 35, 40
Heberden, Revd Edward 36
Heberden Society 17, 18, 26, 29, 33-35, 39, 40, 42, 55, 61, 62, 73, 102
Heberden, William 36, 39, 102
Hench, Philip 14, 22, 35, 41, 54, 76
hepatolenticular degeneration (see Wilson's disease)
hermadactyl 83
Higgs, Sydney L 40
Hill, Leslie 30, 43
Holbrook, Dr Paul 72
Hollander, Joseph Lee 85
Horder, Sir Thomas, later Lord 7, 27-29, 31, 33, 37, 40, 48-50, 54, 68, 69, 99
Horder Homes 18, 68, 69
Hospital Saturday Fund 51
Hospital Saving Association 51
Howell, Victor 33
Howitt, Frank 34, 35, 39, 40, 45, 49, 50, 54, 93
Hutchinson, Sir Robert 31
hydrocortisone 85
hydroxychloroquine 88
hyperuricaemia 91
hypoxanthine 91

'independent trusts' (see NHS)
Indocid 84
indomethacin 84, 87
inflammatory joint disease 79
International Congress on Physical Medicine 76
International Congress of Rheumatology 56
International League Against Rheumatism (ILAR) 12, 13, 65, 71
International Federation of Physical Medicine 49, 50
International Research Centre for Rheumatic Disease, Amsterdam 11

International Society of Medical Hydrology (ISMH) 9, 11
Archives of Medical Hydrology 9, 11
Irgapyrin 86, 87

Jaffe, IA 89
Jamieson, Sir Wilson 7, 27
Jansen 9
Jennings, GH 22, 84
Jimenez-Diaz, C 90
John, Admiral Sir Casper 69
Jones, Sir Robert 23
Journal of Physical Medicine and Industrial Hygiene (see BAPM)
Journal of Rheumatology and Rehabilitation (see BAPM)
Judet acrylic head 23
Jung 14

Kahlmeter 9
Keizersgracht, Amsterdam 11
Kekwick, Professor Alan
Kellgren, Jonas H 41, 63
Kendall, Edward Calvin 14, 22, 35, 41
Kennedy, Mathilde 65
Kennedy Research Institute of Rheumatology 33, 65
Kent, Duchess of (see Marina, Princess)
Kiernander, Basil 45, 49
Kindersley, Charles 30
Klemperer, Paul 23, 56
Korman 9
Kovacs, Richard 76
Koytes Estate, Watford 67
Kraus, Hans 76
Krusen, Frank 49, 50, 76

La Ligue Contre le Rhumatism 42
  Acta Rheumatologica 9, 10-12, 18
Lancefield, RC 22, 83
Lancet 10
Laventhal, Walter 30
LE cell 23
lead palsy 3
Lennep 9
Lenoch, Professor Frantisek 6

Von Leyden 18
Lilly 23
Light, Sydney 76
  World Directory of Physical Medicine Specialists 76
Living with Disability (see Rusk, Howard)
London Hospital 18, 65, 99
Lowman, Edward 76
Lyme disease (see polyarthritis)
Lyme Green Hall, Macclesfield 67

Macleod, Ian 50, 55
McCarty, Daniel 22
McConkey, B 90
McEwen, Currier 73
Maini, Professor RN 18
manipulation 19
Margaret, Princess 69
Marina, Princess 3, 33, 36, 56
Mary, Queen 34
Mason, Michael 18, 33, 65, 100
Mathilde and Terence Kennedy Charitable Trust 65
medical audit (see NHS)
Medical Society of London 49
Mennell, JB 18, 48, 49, 69
Mepacrin 88
methotrexate 90
Michotte 14
Middlesex Hospital, London 28, 35, 65
mithramycin 79
mitral stenosis 83
mixed connective tissue disease 79
Mixter, WJ 78
Moll, John 35
  The Heberden Society 35, 40
Moncrieff, Alan 31
Moore vitallium ball and socket 23
Moran, Lord 31
Myocrisin 83

Naegleriae fowleri 6
National Advisory Arthritis and Rheumatism Council 72
National Ankylosing Spondylitis Society (NASS) 69
National Arthritis and Rheumatism Institute 72
National Back Pain Association 18, 69
  Talk Back 69
National Health Service (NHS) 6-8, 35, 49, 51-63, 67, 74, 75, 93, 94, 96, 99
  independent trusts 53
  medical audit 97
  'opting out' 52, 53
National Institute of Arthritis and Metabolic Disease (NIAMD) 72, 73
Nelson, Selwyn 14
Nesterov, Professor 18
Neuberger, Albert 42
Nissen, JS 34
nitrogen mustard 90
non-steroidal anti-inflammatory drugs (NSAIDs) 23, 85-88, 90
Nuffield, Lord 68

O'Malley, EE 93
Ogilvie, Hon Angus 68
Oliver, William 1
'opting out' (see NHS)
osteoarthritis 95
osteomalacia 79
osteomyelitis 23
osteoporosis 23, 79
Osgood, Robert 23
osmic acid 90
Osmond-Clarke, Sir Henry 93
overlap syndromes 79
oxyphenylbutazone 87

Page, Francis 88
Paget's disease 79
Pan American League Against Rheumatism (PANLAR) 14
Papworth Village Settlement 50
Paraplegic International Olympic Games 67
Parry, Kit Wynn 45
Patterson, 'Pat' 39, 43
Pemberton, Ralph 9, 10, 12, 14, 71
D penicillamine 89
penicillin 83, 84, 91
peptic ulceration 83
Peto Place Red Cross Clinic for Rheumatic Disease 11, 28, 34, 35, 39, 43

phenylbutazone 84, 86, 87, 91
phlebo-thrombosis 87
phthisis 88
physiatry 74-76
Physical Medicine Congress 9
Pletney, Professor 12
poliomyelitis 23
Polley 14, 22
polyarthritis 79, 80, 90, 97
  Lyme disease 79
polymyalgia rheumatica
  syndrome 22, 79
Porritt, Lord Arthur 33
Powell, Sir Richard 69
prednisolone 85
probenecid 84, 91
pseudo-gout 78
psoriatic arthropathy 97
pyrophosphate arthropathy 78

radiotherapy 22
Ragan, Charles 42
Rawson Convalescent Centre 4
Ray, Matthew 34, 35, 37, 40, 49
relapsing polychondritis 79
*Reports on the Incidence of the
  Rheumatic Diseases (1924-28)*
  (see Glover, Alison)
rheumatic fever 21, 22, 25, 72, 77, 83
Rheumatism Reviews (see AACR)
rheumatoid arthritis 1, 22, 25, 30, 42, 85, 87, 88
*Rheumatology and Physical
  Medicine* (see BARR)
Rheumatology and Rehabilitation
  (see BARR)
Robinson, Sidney 30
Rolfe, Mrs Neville 68
Rolleston, Sir Humphrey 31
Romans 1, 3, 4
Rose 23
Royal Bath Hospital, Harrogate 4
Royal College of Physicians 21, 29, 31, 35, 49, 55, 102
  Diploma in Medical Rehabilitation 62
  Diploma of Physical Medicine 31, 49, 61, 102

Royal College of Surgeons 49, 56
Royal Devonshire Hospital 3
Royal Leamington Spa 4
Royal Mineral Water Hospital
  (Min) (see Bath)
Royal National Hospital for
  Rheumatic Diseases (see Bath)
Royal Society of Medicine (RSM)
  31, 37, 42, 100
Royal United Hospital, Bath (see
  Bath)
Rundles 22
Rusk, Howard 76
  Text Book of Rehabilitation 76

Sadler, Miss 69
salicylate 22, 83, 84, 90, 91
Savage, Oswald 17, 65
Schmidt 9
sciatica 3, 78
Scudamore 25
Seegmiller 22
Selye, Hans 22, 41, 56
Sharpe, GC 79
Shrewsbury, Earl of 3
Shulman LE 79
Sitaj 6, 22
Slocumb 14, 22
Smart, Sir Morton 18, 48, 49
Smith-Peterson vitallium cup 23
Society of Physical Therapy 11
sodium aurothiomalate 83
South East Asian, Pacific and
  Australasian League
  (SEAPAL) 14
Spender, Dr J 1
Spinal Injuries Centre, Stoke
  Mandeville 50, 66, 67
spondylitis 21, 23
Spondylitis Society 68
sports medicine 80
St Bartholomew's Hospital,
  London 3, 18, 21, 26, 28, 29, 40, 65
St John's and St Elizabeth's
  Hospital, London 4, 43
St Stephen's Hospital, London 4, 43
St Thomas's Hospital, London 3, 18, 28, 62, 63, 69

Stanley, Sir Arthur 34
  Arthur Stanley Institute 34, 35, 41
Stanton-Woods, Sir Robert 18, 48
Star and Garter Home, London 67
Stecher, Robert 41
steroids 22, 91
Stockman 25
Storey, Dr GO 50
Strasser 9
Strathpeffer 10
Streptococcus viridans 22, 83
stroke 94
sulphapyridine 90
sulphinpyrazone 84, 91
sulphonamides 83
sulphasalazine 89, 90
systemic lupus erythematosus 78, 88
Systemic lupus groups 68
Svartz, Nana 89

Talbott, JH 22, 84
Talk Back (see National Back Pain Association)
Tedder, Lord 50
Tegner, William 39, 99
Text Book of Rehabilitation (see Rusk, Howard)
Thompson, Miss Tatham 9
Trust for Relief of the Poor 4
Tuberculosis of bone and joint 4, 21-23, 42, 83
Tunbridge, Sir Ronald 40
Tweedsmuir, Lord 18, 56, 68

ultra violet radiation 18
United States Public Health Service 72

urate 84
uricosuric 22, 84, 91

Victoria, Queen 4

Waaler 23
Wall, Lord 69
Walthard, Professor 50
Watson-Jones, Sir Reginald 93
Wells 22
Wesson, Arthur 39
West London Rheumatology Department 5
Westminster, Duke of 68
Whitby, Sir Lionel 36
Wilkinson, Professor 24
Willcox, Sir William 31, 33
Wilson's disease 89
Wimshurst machine 18, 21
Winternitz 18
Wolfson Research Centre, Bath (see Bath)
Woolf, Dr Douglas 68, 69
World Directory of Physical Medicine Specialists (see Light, Sydney)
World Rheumatism Year 15
Wright, Dr Beric 69
Wright Fleming Institute of Microbiology, London 42

xanthine oxidase 22, 84, 91

Yeomans 43
yttrium 90

World Health Organisation (WHO) 15

Ziff, Morris 42
Zyloprim 84

Addendum

In a subject that is so rapidly developing, such as rheumatology, its history requires updating virtually every year. In 1991, since this book has been in production, the BSR has reviewed its consultant training recommendations. Research, though important, need not include a full-time period. General medicine should continue, possibly with rotation with other specialties. Training should certainly include some experience in rehabilitation medicine.

These recommendations are completely in harmony with the experience of the past outlined in this book.